FROM THE FLYING SQUAD TO

INVESTIGATING WAR CRIMES

To the memory of my beloved grandfather (Peter Sneddon) and my mother Ann; my sister Irene; my long-suffering wife Sheila, who selflessly permitted me the time and space to travel afar and complete the quests set before me; as well as my two wonderful daughters Lorna and Ceri, all of whom helped me to become the man I am. I'm happy and very proud to call them my family.

FROM THE FLYING SQUAD TO

INVESTIGATING WAR CRIMES

EXPLOITS OF A FORMER SCOTLAND YARD DETECTIVE

From Containment of an Outbreak of Epizootic Lymphangitis in Fife to
Genocide Investigations in the Balkans

RON TURNBULL

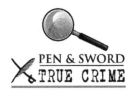

PEN & SWORD
TRUE CRIME

First published in Great Britain in 2019 by
PEN AND SWORD TRUE CRIME
an imprint of
Pen and Sword Books Ltd
Yorkshire – Philadelphia

Hardback ISBN: 978 1 52675 866 8
Paperback ISBN: 978 1 52676 647 2

Typeset in Times New Roman 11.5/14 by
Aura Technology and Software Services, India
Printed and bound in the UK
by TJ International, Padstow, Cornwall, PL28 8RW

Pen & Sword Books Ltd incorporates the imprints of Pen & Sword
Archaeology, Atlas, Aviation, Battleground, Discovery,
Family History, History, Maritime, Military, Naval, Politics, Railways,
Select, Social History, Transport, True Crime, Claymore Press,
Frontline Books, Leo Cooper, Praetorian Press, Remember When,
Seaforth Publishing and Wharncliffe.

For a complete list of Pen & Sword titles please contact
PEN & SWORD BOOKS LIMITED
47 Church Street, Barnsley, South Yorkshire, S70 2AS, England
E-mail: enquiries@pen-and-sword.co.uk
Website: www.pen-and-sword.co.uk

Or
PEN AND SWORD BOOKS
1950 Lawrence Rd, Havertown, PA 19083, USA
E-mail: Uspen-and-sword@casematepublishers.com
Website: www.penandswordbooks.com

Contents

Introduction vii

Foreword ix

Chapter 1   Goodbye Grandad 1

Chapter 2   The Early Days 9

Chapter 3   An Embryonic Police Career 14

Chapter 4   Outward Bound in Burghead on the Moray Firth 23

Chapter 5   Fife Constabulary's First PC 600 27

Chapter 6   Dealing with my First Dead Body 34

Chapter 7   Accused of Theft 38

Chapter 8   Disillusioned of Fife 42

Chapter 9   Time to Move On 49

Chapter 10   Hendon it is then 53

Chapter 11   Balham: A New Beginning 54

Chapter 12   The Sweeney Days 68

Chapter 13   Promotion: Onwards and Upwards 76

Chapter 14   The 'Maltese Mafia' 81

Chapter 15   Back to Normal 87

Chapter 16   Recalled to Flying Squad Duties 96

Chapter 17   Blags 'r' Us 107

Chapter 18   Life after the Flying Squad 113

Chapter 19   Laboratory Liaison Officer 115

Chapter 20   Beaten, Raped and Left to Die in Brixton 125

Chapter 21   Teapot 1 129

Chapter 22   Crime Scene Examination on Wimbledon Common 131

Chapter 23   Who Dares Wins 139

Chapter 24   Political Assassination in Sri Lanka 141

Chapter 25   Provisional Irish Republican Army (PIRA) Bombs
              a Bus in Aldwych 147

Chapter 26   Bosnia Calling 151

Chapter 27   The Village of Cerska in
              Bosnia and Herzegovina 158

Chapter 28   Vukovar Hospital in Croatia 165

Chapter 29   The British Forensic Team: Kosovo 1999 170

Chapter 30   The Village of Celina in Kosovo 176

Chapter 31   The Village of Velika Kruša in Kosovo 179

Chapter 32   Lapsed Security 181

Chapter 33   Miscellany 183

Chapter 34   Health & Safety 185

Chapter 35   Political Murder in the Republic of Zambia 188

Chapter 36   The BFT and I Return to Kosovo: 2000 192

Chapter 37   The Start of Another Career in the United Nations 200

Chapter 38   All Work and No Play 203

Chapter 39   Beware of Mines 209

Chapter 40   Fatal Bombing of the UN HQ Building
              in Baghdad 211

Chapter 41   UNICEF in Sudan 216

Chapter 42   Historical Enquiries Team (HET), part of the
              Police Service Northern Ireland (PSNI) 226

Chapter 43   Remembering Srebrenica 230

Index 233

Introduction

So many times over the years in my various and varied careers members of my family, many friends and peers have urged me with the words: 'Ron, there's got to be a book in you.' I pushed such thoughts away time and time again because I was either too busy, or I didn't think there would be an audience that would be interested in, never mind want to read about my exploits, or maybe the truth was that I just couldn't be bothered.

Autobiography is a special type of biography that follows its own rules and may vary substantially in content, style, length and purpose. It may concentrate on the purely professional aspects of one's life or dwell on the familial, political and social atmosphere of your time and describe in detail your qualities and fallibilities as well as, hopefully in a light-hearted way, those of colleagues. The structure of such a book can be a series of unrelated anecdotes or simply document chronologically and dispassionately the life experiences of an individual who carried out the duties related to his/her job in a competent way.

Eventually, as I faced my seventh decade, I came to the realization that a reasonable compromise would be to pen some of my more memorable personal and professional challenges and achievements. This was not so much for public consumption but to provide my two wonderful daughters with a heartfelt written record so that they would come to know more about, and hopefully better understand, where their errant dad was, as well as what and with whom he was engaged, on the many occasions in their lives when I probably should have spent more time with them as they were growing up. Like many of my generation, I have sincere regrets for not asking my late mother, or grandfather for that matter, many more questions about their lives and personal trials and tribulations when they were still around. Furthermore, by compiling this missive, my own two wee worthy grandsons Harris and Jack will have access to a point of reference in which I will have hopefully described some of the many important aspects of the social history surrounding my lifetime if or when they want to know more about their grandad and his generation.

Having given myself a green light to undertake this mission, I'm more than aware that there might be inaccuracies due to lapses or failings in my memory. However, to quote that great comedy film star Groucho Marx, I'm not going to let the truth spoil a good story!

So, with fingers crossed, here goes…

Ron Turnbull
(Retired at last)

Foreword

The following is a wonderful account of detective work by an outstanding practitioner of the artisan craft. It contains exciting experiences told clearly, but also lessons for everyone who criticizes in general terms the dedicated public servants who make a less than perfect system work for society, those critics who find misconduct in every contested policing interaction.

I was fortunate to serve closely with Ron Turnbull during nearly forty years at New Scotland Yard. We first met while serving on different teams of the Flying Squad, a prestige, specialist posting confronting serious thieves, robbers, drug dealers, organized and disorganized criminals. Our joy was in the hunt, arrest and conviction of these predators on society. Ron describes his journey from Fife to this undergrowth of civilization in London in detail and his role in a highly specialized squad.

Our next set of adventures together were with the Flying Squad again, this time some years later at an outstation in South London as part of the Robbery Squad (a transfiguration of the Flying Squad). Though tasked with dealing with armed robbery, we could sometimes wangle our investigative way into other kinds of violent and organized crime. Ron is modest about his role here. I was present when an Old Bailey High Court Red Judge said in Ron's presence to an armed robbery defendant that the only reason he was there to be sentenced was because 'Detective Sergeant Turnbull and Detective Constable XXX did not shoot you dead as they would have been perfectly entitled to do.' The judge went on to commend the two officers for their skills and outstanding courage.

The next time our paths crossed was in intelligence where we were involved in staff work and some practical applications; Ron was tackling the complex protection of some of our most important but vulnerable informers. From there he went into another aspect of intelligence, this time the public outreach for information via Crimestoppers at its early introduction in the UK.

The last adventures we had together were at the nexus of forensic science and counter-terrorism. One dark evening I asked his permission to enter a fatal terrorism crime scene; although I was the Senior Officer present, Ron was the professional, the crime scene manager and therefore in charge. In time he moved on to his role in investigating international war crimes and genocide and we would meet up once a year for a Flying Squad reunion.

His book is, then, a description of Ron's many roles. His account of multiple aspects of policing, it contains detailed descriptions of detective tactics and investigative strategy, a record of what he did and why he did it. He includes everything from international inquiries to street crime in London and all in between.

This is a book I have longed for and begged him to write. I wanted to be able to cite Ron's experiences to my Masters and Doctoral students in greater detail. Highly professional, a leader, a skilled tactician, a master of his craft, his account makes a mockery of the simplistic negative politicized narratives of twenty-first-century policing. This is the antidote to the misdescriptions of so many politicians, seeking to justify austerity, some critical but ignorant academics and some, but not all, journalists (Bob Chesshyre is an exception; he wrote a valuable long article about Ron in the *Sunday Telegraph* in 2002 and also encouraged him to write this book). It is an exact, definitive, lively narrative of what the best public servants, those hard-working detectives, experienced in a complex variety of tasks, some deeply unpleasant yet hugely rewarding. Thank you Ron, and all those like you. The very best of simply the best.

Professor Emeritus John G.D. Grieve
CBE, QPM, BA(Hons), MPhil, HonDL.
Former Deputy Assistant Commissioner at New Scotland Yard
London, November 2018

Chapter 1

Goodbye Grandad

I never got to see my grandfather's body laid out after he died, nor had any opportunity for private words with him before his burial, which haunted me in a curious way for many years afterwards. This may have been due to my perceived youthfulness in the eyes of two of my mother's three older brothers who even objected to me being a pallbearer at his funeral, preferring their own sons to carry out this very personal function. Mum, although very much the baby of the family, could be quite resolute so she fought her corner with her siblings in this matter, ensuring that I did officiate as one of grandad's pallbearers, along with my uncles and cousins. This was massively important to me because of the love and great respect I had for him. After all, he had been living with my family for the last few years of his life so I'd had much more contact with him than his sons and his other grandchildren. Or was it something more sinister?

My mum had been in an unhappy marriage in the late 1940s and as a result was living apart from her husband while divorce proceedings were in progress. She had a short love affair with a co-worker at the Royal Naval Dockyard in Rosyth, near Dunfermline, Fife where she was employed along with quite a number of other ladies painting the hulls and upper deck areas on naval vessels. Imagine going to work every day to paint warships using a wide brush on the end of a very long pole...and always in battleship grey. Yours truly was the unplanned and unforeseen result of this union. Having a child born out of wedlock, or to use the local phraseology of that time, 'born on the other side of the sheets' was not at all easy for the mother. There was a social stigma attached in those days. Society tended to look down on the mother and sometimes the bastard child too. When she declared her pregnancy to her father, stating that she wanted to keep the baby (her mother had died several years previously), even he told her: 'You've made your bed, now you'll have to lie in it.' Grandad allowed mum to move in with him to reduce her expenditure and help her through the hard times to come. I was born in his house.

In hindsight I'm of the opinion that her older brothers were more than rather standoffish. They rarely came visiting, as I recall. Occasionally one or other of my aunts would pop in to visit grandad and make a wee fuss of me. It may seem strange to the reader, but I knew nothing of this until I was well into my 20s and embarking on a career of my own in the police. Mum eventually succumbed to my questions about my biological or 'real father' after I'd picked up on a few conversations within her family that led me to believe that I was adopted. She broke down and insisted that she would only tell me about my origins if I promised not to seek out my biological father. She knew that as a policeman I would be in a better position than most to do so. I agreed to this deal and never did seek him out, although I came close to it a couple of times. Imagine how much pocket money he owed me!

I've always been immensely proud of my mum. On reflection over the years I've thought it was pretty cool that when I was a youngster there would have been Royal Navy battleships sailing around the world which she had helped to paint. More seriously, for her to decide to raise me on her own with all the trials, tribulations and innuendo she knew that could bring was truly courageous but, overall, a most loving thing to do. I could never thank her enough for giving me life. I did all I could throughout her life to make her proud of her 'wee Ronnie'. I hope I succeeded in that endeavour.

I vividly remember that late-night knock on our front door in early December 1966, my mother's voice emitting a sorrowful and repetitious 'No, No' and 'Ronnie, it's your Granfaither' as she sobbed deeply and cried over being told of the death of her beloved father. Mum had personally cared for him in our home for many years before medical necessity convinced both of them that it would be much better for all concerned if he were admitted to hospital, which we knew actually meant hospice. This advice she heeded with some reluctance, but never really accepted it as the best solution. I recall seeing the not unattractive ginger-haired policewoman (WPC) and her younger male colleague trying to console my mum outside our front door. In her shocked state she had omitted to invite the officers in, so when I appeared from my bedroom they were all three crowded into the small hallway of our council flat in Lochgelly, then still a coal-mining town in Fife, central Scotland.

Fife, also known as The Kingdom, is the county depicted in the dog's head shape jutting out into the North Sea on maps displaying the east coast of Scotland, situated between the estuaries (or firths) of the magnificent Forth and Tay Rivers and the cities and sea ports of Edinburgh and Dundee respectively. The only claim to fame, or should I say notoriety, that Lochgelly possessed to my knowledge at that time in the minds of generations of schoolchildren was that a local garage, G.W. Dicks & Sons, produced the infamous strap or belt known in old Scots as the tawse or taws; a leather strap cut into strips at the end. This was unique to Scottish education and was used as a form of corporal punishment by sadistic teachers upon the hands of their unfortunate pupils in the days before this Draconian weapon of torture was quite rightly banned from use in Scottish schools.

I was taught at one stage by a Religious Instruction teacher, a man of the cloth for Christ's sake (no pun intended), nicknamed by the pupils as 'Holy Joe', who had three of these straps of varying thickness, which he named after three of Jesus' disciples. If you were unfortunate enough to transgress in his classroom he allowed you to choose your own means of punishment …thank you very much. Given his profession and calling, I thought this bizarre in the extreme, which may go a long way to explain my agnostic, if not atheistic, view of religion to this day. Obviously most of us chose the most slender version of strap, but this was a mistake because it had three strips cut into the end that stung like hell when he whipped it across your poor palm.

Lochgelly was a grey, drab, almost characterless town showing the beginnings of decay and commercial dilapidation of the 1960s as the surrounding coal mines were closing down with regular monotony and the coal miners, who had neither known nor probably considered any other occupation all of their working lives, were being made redundant and placed on the dole. Everything and almost everyone appeared to me to be grey and depressing. It's not the prettiest part of the otherwise beautiful county of Fife which is home to the world-renowned town of St Andrews with its majestic and historic golf courses and beautiful inviting sandy beaches, as well as the magnificent university buildings of this truly noble old regal town.

In this same part of Fife, known locally as the East Neuk, the visitor will find many picturesque fishing villages with romantic names such as St Monans, Pittenweem, Crail, Lundin Links and Anstruther, all of which have something special to offer the discerning traveller. The hill walks along the coastline facing the Firth of Forth are something to behold, regardless of the season or the ever-changeable weather, from where the Isle of May can be seen on a clear day as you look towards the city of Edinburgh on the south shore of the firth. May Isle is a National Nature Reserve managed by Scottish National Heritage which provides much-needed protection for grey seals, puffins and many other species of migratory seabirds.

The closest largish town to Lochgelly is Dunfermline, the former capital of Scotland and one-time seat of the kings of Scotland, especially the dynasty of Robert the Bruce, which sits proudly nearby. Dunfermline was the birthplace of the great philanthropist Andrew Carnegie who accrued a fortune in America. With its magnificent public park known as The Glen and many architecturally interesting and impressive public buildings built through Carnegie's funding, it is drenched in history. It is also the footballing home of the 'Pars' as Dunfermline Athletic Football Club is known locally. Apparently this is derived from the word 'paralytic', which describes how the locals viewed their team's soccer abilities in the past. A bit unfair, methinks.

On the east side of Lochgelly, about the same distance away as Dunfermline, is the 'Lang Toun' of Kirkcaldy, notorious for the odorous smells that once wafted from the many tall factory chimneys of its main industry in bygone days involving linoleum production. This is also a town steeped in history with its own splendid public Ravenscraig Park and many miles of white sandy beaches along the embankment. It is also the home of Raith Rovers Football Club, of which former Prime Minister Gordon Brown claimed to be a fan and regular attendee at their home games. The truth is, however, I neither know nor have heard of anyone who has actually seen him there.

I'm willing to admit to having read all of the highly-acclaimed and extremely popular author Ian Rankin's 'Inspector Rebus' crime novels that are set in Edinburgh, Scotland's magnificent capital city, which is about half an hour's car drive south of Fife across the Forth Road Bridge. Ian Rankin is a fellow Fifer and like myself a former pupil of Beath High School, Cowdenbeath. In one of his books, I think *Dead Souls*, we find the main character Detective Inspector Rebus recount alighting from a train in Cardenden, Fife and how desperately drab and dilapidated this former coal mining village, similar in many ways and positioned very close to Lochgelly, was. Another author, Kate Atkinson, in *Behind the Scenes at the Museum* went further and wrote:

> Once I caught a train to Cardenden by mistake… When we reached Cardenden we got off and waited for the next train back to Edinburgh. I was very tired and if Cardenden had looked more promising, I think I would have simply stayed there. If you've ever been to Cardenden, you'll know how bad things must have been.

A trifle harsh perhaps, but this for me also summed up drab old Lochgelly at the time.

The two police officers gave me the impression that because my grandad had been in the hospice, financed and provided by the National Coal Board (NCB) for former coal miners, for some time and was in his mid-80s, his death was to be expected. The WPC repeatedly said that he'd died peacefully and without pain. Even then, in my naivety and grief, I recall thinking: 'How does she know? How does anybody know?'

I was also aware of a growing personal anger that I could not properly explain for a long time afterwards. Courteous yet perfunctory and obviously intent on moving on to far more serious and demanding constabulary matters, the officers asked if we wanted to attend the local police station to use the telephone. They rightly assumed that we didn't have a phone installed in our house, which was not unusual at that time. Of our group of friends and family I think only one possessed a telephone then. When I declined their kind offer, the WPC wrote down and passed me the hospice telephone number and advised me to make contact later in the morning. She then asked if I was okay and able to look after my mother. I was all of 18 years young. My step-father Tam, also a coal miner, was at work. The officer then noticed my uniform cap hanging in the hallway above my police issue greatcoat, the latter with the emblem sewn on each shoulder declaring the wearer to be a police cadet, while the cap displayed the same silver metal Fife Constabulary badge as the one adorning her own be-capped head, bearing the Scottish Police motto *Semper Vigilo* ('Always Watchful') under a thistle design shining forth from the front of the light blue band (see photo plate section).

Her unwittingly patronizing attitude immediately changed and she began to ask me questions relating to our shared profession such as where I was stationed, did I know officer so-and-so, and when would I graduate to the full force, all while Mum sobbed away beside me. In fairness, she then kindly added that if there was anything they could do to help, I could contact them anytime during their night shift. She then politely and abruptly made her exit, followed by her apprentice and, possibly mute, colleague.

More than once during my almost thirty-five-year police career that followed I recalled this day. This was partly because I was very close to my grandad or, to use the old Fife vernacular, my 'Di' (pronounced 'dye'). It's believed that this is a derivative of the Spanish/French word 'Grandee' meaning 'of great personage' and is a leftover from bygone days when the capital of Scotland was Dunfermline and of course French and Spanish would be spoken in the royal court of the Robert the Bruce monarchy. Much later, when relatives of murder victims asked to see their loved ones at an appropriate time during police enquiries, I felt a strong empathy for them to be accorded this right, mainly I believe because I would have liked to have been given the opportunity to talk to and say a form of farewell to my very own beloved Di.

He had been a self-employed 'shot-firer' who for all of his hard-working life was engaged in the mainly undersea coal mines of Fife, ably abetted by his three sons for their entire arduous working lives too. Their job was to manually drill holes into the coalface and insert dynamite in order to blow the coal seams out for the miners to grade and retrieve the rough coal; the latter a process known rather innocuously as 'brushing'. This rough coal was then taken up to the surface of the colliery by small-gauge trains comprising engines known as 'pugs' pulling open carriages known as 'bogies' along narrow rail tracks. Ton after heavy ton of coal was removed in this manner, eventually to fuel the furnaces of heavy industry, propel the much larger steam trains and engines of the era or simply heat the many local homes.

By April 1948 when mum produced her little surprise package, namely me, Di was a retired old chap living in a typical miner's cottage in a row in the village of Hill of Beath named Engine Row, but locally referred to as Pug Row, long since bulldozed into oblivion. He was always to be found, regardless of the weather, in the miners' ubiquitous Fife cloth 'bunnet' (cloth cap), his favoured waistcoats with watch chain displayed proudly, and highly-shined and well-cobbled boots. He enjoyed the odd game of dominoes and a pipe of tobacco accompanied by a few drinks in the local so-called miners' welfare club. I can still recall the smell of his pipe tobacco, Heath Brown Flake brand, which he mixed with a plug of chewing tobacco. Pretty pungent and potent stuff, I can tell you. He also seemed to have a limitless supply of Pan Drops which were strong mint sweets he often shared with me and to which I'm still almost addicted.

Occasionally I was allowed to accompany him on these trysts with his old coal miner pals. I was allowed to sit quietly alongside them, duly supplied with a soft drink and a packet of crisps, watching them play dominoes. I imagined them akin to gunslingers from the old 'B' cowboy movies, because at the start of their evening they would buy a couple of half pints of ale plus a quart bottle of whisky, which came with two shot glasses. This they carried along with a box of dominoes to their favourite table over by the bay window of the local miners' welfare institute, just like ageing cowboys setting up a card table a bit out of step with the progress of time.

Di used to regale me with tales of the hazards, and oft times horrors, of working below ground, and the near-disaster situations he and my uncles had experienced. He also rallied forth about the pious, aloof and uncaring attitudes of many private colliery managers of that time in the days before the NCB unified the collieries and the rights and health and safety considerations of the miners were drastically reviewed and belatedly improved. These were times when miners would have to endure working their entire shift in filthy salt water in the wet pits under the seabed of the Firth of Forth for literally only a few pence more per day, providing the manager approved that it was worth the additional payment, of course. The yardstick for this was that the water level had to be up to their knees during their entire shift, would you believe.

Little wonder then that the famous Welsh politician Aneurin 'Nye' Bevan worked relentlessly on behalf of these socially abused and disadvantaged workmen at that time. His wife, Jenny Wren, also a prominent socialist politician of that era, originated from this part of Fife so she would have had first-hand knowledge of the grim manner in which these men were treated.

While I was still of primary school age Tam was badly injured in a coal mine roof cave-in, or 'fall' as the miners called it, which left him with a serious back problem. As a result, after several months of not too good medical treatment or physiotherapy he was deemed unable to return to coal-mining work. At that time our family resided in a house belonging to the NCB from which we were given notice to leave because Tam was no longer to be an NCB employee. There was no alternative local council housing available so we were forced to rent a caravan on a residential site just outside the small village of Townhill near Dunfermline for about a year. I remember it always felt cold and naturally quite cramped inside the caravan and the toilet and shower facilities were extremely basic. Interestingly the site had been a Fleet Air Arm station supporting and protecting the nearby naval dockyard at Rosyth during the Second World War and was occupied by around 100 Wrens (Women's Royal Navy personnel) as well as 1,000 sailors and airmen and had been named HMS *Waxwing*.

Chapter 2

The Early Days

My working life began at 16 years of age when I left Beath High School in Cowdenbeath (another Fife coal-mining town) sporting fewer 'O' levels than I'd hoped for. On a week when I wasn't sitting any 'O'-level exams a few school chums and I decided to 'bunk off' or, to be precise, play truant and spend the time in the summer countryside. Unfortunately for us the school authorities rightly suspected that we were up to no good so letters arrived at our addresses for the attention of our parents asking why we hadn't attended school. My mum was devastated. Her 'wee Ronnie' couldn't have played truant, could he? I was really ashamed, so humbly apologized and admitted my fall from grace. We were all summoned to the headmaster's office where the formidable head, Mr Eadie, administered six of the belt to each of us, which was painful. Worse than that though, was that he'd read in my school careers file that I intended to make the police my career. While giving me a dressing-down he emphasized that my deceit to my mother and my school were not the values expected in a police officer. He ended up by telling me to buck up my ideas or I'd never make anything of my life. That really hurt, but stuck with me for the rest of my life. Much as I'd have liked to have continued my education and possibly enter university, the reality was that I needed to earn my keep to help support the family. I'd already made a start by becoming a daily newspaper delivery boy and worked on a local farm most weekends.

I'd harboured the notion of becoming a police officer for a few years. In fact, a female friend with whom I attended primary school reminded me a few years ago that I'd talked of becoming a policeman even as early as then. My great-grandfather had been a police constable (PC) in a small burgh police force in Kincardine which is situated on the Fife border with Stirling and Clackmannanshire for some years before eventually returning to coal-mining because his police salary was insufficient for him to maintain his family. Di was actually born in a police house in that burgh in August 1882 which then incorporated the village of Tulliallan where many years later (1954 in fact) the Scottish Police College would be built, which I would attend. By the way, Tulliallan in Gaelic means 'beautiful knoll' but I don't recall seeing such a knoll there.

My favourite cousin Irene who often baby-sat me apparently to allow mum to go out to work and have the occasional night out had married a Glaswegian chap named Ian Campbell who was then a PC in Fife. Because of the lack of opportunities for promotion he subsequently transferred to the then City of Glasgow police where he eventually retired as a chief inspector in their Command and Control Centre. While he was still in the Fife Constabulary I spent some of my summer school holidays with them and their sons in their police house in the ornate village of Kingsbarns just outside St Andrews, and became more and more interested in a police career as Ian gave me an insight into rural police work.

I recall with fondness him telling my mum that after his first date with Irene when he was doing his National Service in the RAF and she was working in a clothing factory that he'd told his mother that he'd just met the woman he would marry. 'How do you know?' his mum asked, to which he replied: 'Because she has lovely eyes, just like our collie's.' What a compliment. Sure enough they did marry, produced four fine sons and remained happily married until Ian's untimely death in 2013. Over the years Ian was to become the father figure I never had as well as my mentor and confidant and sort of big brother. I sorely miss his sage counsel and friendship, but above all I miss him.

Ian suggested I consider becoming a police cadet, so with that in mind I decided to apply to the largest and I would say the best police force in the country, despatching a letter to the commissioner of the Metropolitan Police, New Scotland Yard, London, SW1. My handful of 'O' levels were sufficient for entry and I knew of no medical condition that would debar me. The British police still had a height restriction in those days, generally 5ft 10in in Scotland, but as I stood 5ft 11in tall the Met's bar of 5ft 8in was no problem. I was requested to attend for a medical examination and interview at one of the Met's recruiting centres in Borough High Street, London so off I toddled, full of hope, anticipation and excitement; however:

- Woe and behold, I failed the medical!
- I was classified as underweight for my age and height!
- I was absolutely shattered!
- My perceived future was in absolute ruins!

However, a recruiting officer kindly informed me that in all other respects I was acceptable, but as they had a limited intake the Met couldn't offer me a cadet post at this time. He advised me to build up some muscle and then apply again at a later date.

I returned home, to say the least a tad down-beaten, but resolved to get a job as soon as possible in order to tide me over until I could have another crack at joining the police but also to see what life had in store for me. I obtained a trainee factory post with Dunfermline Silk Mills which offered a reasonable wage plus the prospect of a good apprenticeship, possibly culminating in me joining their men's necktie design team in Switzerland. However, that was a long way off. I had to work my way up through the shop floor first. This meant I was assigned to a 'tenter' as a 'grease monkey'. A tenter is the engineer responsible for keeping the looms operating. The shop floor (referred to by the machine operators as 'the shed') consisted of more than 100 looms clattering and bashing away noisily all day long producing many variants of silk cloth from which others would create a plethora of fine goods. The air was filled with choking silk dust and other detritus that doesn't bear thinking about. The so-called air filters and fans were totally inadequate for the task of keeping the dust to an acceptable level. Health and Safety as we know it was not so demanding or prevalent in those days. The operators of these looms, called weavers, were nearly all women and they were most demanding when their looms broke down because while inoperative it cost them hard-earned money.

Being at the bottom of this work ladder, I received a fair bit of stick initially. In order to grease a loom you have to wriggle underneath it and apply light oil to all moveable parts and heavier grease in a grease gun to ensure the numerous grease nipples are kept filled to a prescribed level. This was often, if not always, done while the loom was operating mere inches above your head. Once again, Health and Safety was not at a premium. As you lay on your back, most of your torso was under the loom beneath the wooden pedal brake which ran the entire width of it and on which the weavers would stamp to halt the machinery should they notice anything wrong. You were, shall we say, vulnerable.

On one occasion a weaver renowned for her so-called sense of humour who regularly goaded me about whether I was still a virgin or not decided on a bit of a prank. She and another weaver trod on the brake pedal while I worked away with my grease gun, thus trapping me on the shed floor lying on my back. They then unfastened the flies on my overalls and jeans and applied dollops of grease to my underpants, adding handfuls of silk off-cuts as a decorative parting gift. No doubt a mild teasing form of 'tarring and feathering' in their minds. A few of these female weavers (actually I don't remember there being any male weavers) were, to say the least, a wee bit coarse at times. As laughter and sniggering ensued in that section of the shed, including the tenter, I made myself as decent as I could and hurriedly headed for the gent's loo. I was so embarrassed. The tenter joined me and said it was just a harmless bit of fun and a ritual that all grease monkeys were put through. Just grin and bear it and you'll be fine, he advised. He was probably right under the circumstances. Reluctantly I took his advice and the women's attitude was generally fine from then on. The main characters even eventually apologized. Although such conduct would never be acceptable in today's world, I learned that it was pretty common for apprentices to undergo such treatment then, some a lot worse. Thank goodness we've moved on. I grew to hate the job, however. I hated the shed. I couldn't imagine doing this day after day, no matter what the potential prospects. The basic working conditions were potentially very unhealthy and had become unacceptable to me, so I began to look around for alternative better employment.

I arrived at the mill one morning to learn that there had been a burglary overnight and a large number of tools and specialized equipment had been stolen. Some of these were tools I had been issued by the company. When the local police officers and scenes of crime technicians arrived the place was abuzz with activity and rumour. I was obliged to make a written statement to a CID officer detailing the tools I'd had stolen. After the paperwork was completed I happened to mention to him that I was interested in becoming a police officer; he reported that the Fife Constabulary were increasing their cadet numbers at that time so I should consider applying. After discussing this proposal with my cousin-in-law Ian I did just that. Since being rejected by the Met I'd taken up swimming, cross-country running and gym work so had in fact built myself up a bit. I was more than ready for a proper challenge.

Happy Days. Fife Constabulary offered me a cadet post after a medical and short interview, so after attesting at Police HQ in Kirkcaldy I was assigned to Dunfermline Divisional HQ in Abbey Park Place.

Chapter 3

An Embryonic Police Career

The old Dunfermline Divisional HQ situated in quiet suburban Abbey Park Place was an interesting building. Obviously not built for police purposes, it gave one the impression and feeling of a Victorian country house. The main office could have been a large dining room as it offered a good outlook to what had once probably been a fine expansive garden. Part of this room had been altered to present the 'bowl' or glass-fronted Enquiry Office for the use of the public as they called to report whatever caused them concern or seek police advice. A large wooden table held an assortment of old cardboard files and well-thumbed typed reports in abundance as well as a couple of far from modern heavy metal typewriters, all of which were overseen by the redoubtable Sergeant Andrew S. Scott firmly and without favour.

Sergeant Scott was an amputee, having lost a leg during the Second World War while serving in Bomber Command. He was my boss. The entire unit was headed by a superintendent (Supt) and incorporated a small CID team, an even smaller Women Police section, several Motor Patrol (traffic) officers, a small uniform presence of sergeants and constables under an inspector (Insp), a crime prevention officer as well as a handful of civilian typists and administrators…and now me.

My daily tasks, shared by one other cadet, were to deliver court papers, police prosecution files and letters to the office of the Procurator Fiscal (PF) in the nearby rather majestic Town Hall each morning. The PF is responsible for advising and processing criminal cases on behalf of the police in Scotland. This meant a short walk in uniform through this fine old town a couple of times per day. At the Fiscal's office I was regularly given a cuppa by the female office staff, some of whom reminded me of somewhat prim librarian stereotypes, as I awaited immediate reply to the paperwork I'd delivered. This task was normally repeated in the afternoon.

Back in Abbey Park Place I was responsible for reading through all police and Scottish Office publications, bringing any pertinent data or new operational directions to the attention of Sergeant Scott. This mainly involved a publication named the *Scottish Police Gazette* (SPG) in which suspects wanted for minor offences or more serious crimes or persons simply missing were detailed and, should there be a comment to the effect that he or she 'frequented the Dunfermline area', again I brought this to his attention so that he could alert local officers. The other important aspect of the SPG was ensuring that when arrests had been made or a demise notified of any previous individual circulated, the original SPG was to be corrected/cancelled as appropriate and cross-referenced. Arrests were highlighted in red ink and the deceased in black as instructed by the good sergeant. He would occasionally check them himself which tended to keep one on one's toes. This was really boring and repetitive work, albeit important. The same was required for the *Police Gazette* (PG) which served the same purpose for English and Welsh police forces. That apart, I did a great deal of filing, and of course made the odd cuppa or two.

Speaking of cuppas, the Metropolitan Police was engaged in a recruiting campaign in Scotland at this time and Fife's chief constable had granted their officers permission to do so in our county. A Cadet Kennedy was part of their team and a newspaper article ascribed to him in a Scottish daily newspaper quoted him as saying among other things 'that a cadet's life is more than just making a cup of tea', then he went on to extol the virtues of the Met's cadet training school and the varied sporting opportunities at Hendon Police College. Quite understandable. However, I wasn't inclined to be tolerant when I read it, so for the first and last time I hastily put pen to paper and wrote to the *Daily Record* newspaper in defence of my peers. To my surprise, several days later my letter was published in the 'Letters to the Editor' column as follows:

> I would like to correct any misconceptions which may arise from the article on 'A Metropolitan Police Cadet' of Nov 8th 1966. I am a police cadet in Fife Constabulary and I take exception, probably along with many other police cadets in Scotland, to this statement implying that we are 'skivers lounging about making tea'. Mr Kennedy may have more responsibility than his Scottish counterpart so he should be thankful for the opportunities he has been given and not look down on those less fortunate. Scottish police cadets are

just as capable and make equally good policemen as those in London. If we were offered the same training facilities in Scotland as they have in London we would be only too keen to work and study more. The fault does not lie with the cadets.

I was blissfully unaware of this article when I boarded the bus to Dunfermline and chatted with the conductor. It was standard protocol for police officers (including cadets) when travelling in uniform on Fife's buses to stand on the rear platform with the conductor so as not to take up a seat from the fare-paying public as officers travelled free on Fife's bus service while on duty.

When I arrived at the office Sergeant Scott showed me the article and invited me to read it through. When he saw how surprised and probably shocked I was, he congratulated me for having the guts to stand up for what I thought was an unfair and patronizing comment. A couple of the other office staff said likewise. Just when I was beginning to feel good about my action he added that the Supt wanted to see me as soon as I arrived. Oh dear! Was I about to get drummed out?

Sergeant Scott warned me to only speak when asked to by the Supt and to keep any response short. He then picked up the phone and informed the Insp that I was available. Rather nervously I reported to the Insp's office upstairs, who led me across to the Supt's office. He announced me, then as he closed the door he winked and whispered: 'Don't worry son, he won't bite you.'

Sure enough, the Supt bade me take a seat on the opposite side of his desk (being asked to sit is always a good sign when a subordinate appears before a senior officer), then told me he agreed in principle with my comments in the letter. However, he then carefully explained that I should have sought permission before having a dialogue with the press and impressed upon me the reasoning behind this dictum. After this slight rebuke he put me at ease by informing me that the matter would end with him and went on to talk about my career thus far, with which he was pleased (thank goodness), plus my future prospects in the force. The matter would go no further, he assured me, and as I exited his office I thanked him and confirmed that I wouldn't be writing any more unauthorized letters to anyone and I never did. My mum was really proud though and kept a cut-out copy in her scrapbook to her dying day.

I like to think that perhaps as a result of the Met cadet's comments and my printed response, a further education package was rolled out by Fife HQ in Kirkcaldy for all twelve cadets. We were taught typewriting skills, attended English, Geography and police-related study classes as well as engaging in regular cross-country runs and weekly swimming lessons at a public baths, which included life-saving techniques, by members of the force training unit.

When my admin duties allowed, good old Sergeant Scott occasionally encouraged me to go on foot patrol with a beat PC which was enlightening. Actually experiencing how officers interacted with the public and dealt with matters as they occurred was very instructive, as well as riding along with the Motor Patrol, which was a bit more exhilarating, I have to admit, in the rear of a marked high-performance car. The interface between drivers stopped by these officers was a little less convivial than meeting the public in the street, I noted.

I was taught the now defunct art of manual traffic direction at a fixed point in the High Street which became very busy when the various factories in and around the town closed for the day. Buses, especially double-decker ones filled to capacity, coming up the New Row, a very steep incline, needed to be accorded precedence over other road users. This required some dexterity because the camber of the road here made double-decker buses veer over so that the officer on point duty had to avoid allowing two to pass at the same time because of the danger of getting squashed between them. Duly adorned with my white armlets and whistle, I forgot this on one occasion, resulting in me being spun around between two buses and knocking my cap off, fortunately without injury but with some loss of dignity. I noted a wry smile from the PC which basically said 'Told you so' as he handed me my dusty cap. Ironically only one of the bus drivers stopped to see if I was okay.

I was rather taken with a really pretty WPC in the office at this time. She had long red hair, a lovely figure and an even nicer personality. She chatted to me often, which I think I misjudged somewhat as I privately hoped that maybe when I was appointed as a constable I could ask her out on a date. The very popular Moody Blues pop group held a gig in Dunfermline as part of their UK tour promoting their recent hit *Nights in White Satin* but unfortunately had some of their kit stolen. This lovely WPC reported the crime and when she returned to the office presented me with autographs of the entire band which included the line 'Swap your boots Ron'. What a sweetie. I learned that she played badminton locally so I naively purchased a racket and kit, then joined the club she used only to find that she was dating a PC from our nick and regularly played badminton with him there. End of a potential romance that never was. Onwards and upwards then; on to pastures new.

I was occasionally fortunate enough to attend football matches to assist with crowd control at East End Park, the home of the Pars, which was a real bonus as I'd been a keen fan and supporter for some years. In the same capacity I attended a couple of significant golf tournaments at St Andrews and in August 1966 I was assigned to the complement of Fife officers who policed the formal opening of the Tay Road Bridge. I was linked up with a WPC. We were briefed to ensure that the public did not access the roadway at the Fife end of the bridge during the opening ceremony which was performed by HM The Queen Mother.

In one of my not-too-clever moments I volunteered to assist a dog-handler unit. I've always had a love for our canine buddies. This culminated in a session in a public park where I was suitably dressed in protective clothing and asked to run off and let the German shepherd chase and 'apprehend' me. This I did with gusto and very soon after release the dog brought me down by gripping my heavily padded forearm. The next phase was to carry a blunt knife and turn and threaten the dog with it as it drew near. Again K9 carried out his duty with aplomb. Finally the handler asked me to stop as the dog approached, shout, make loud noises and lunge forward making slashing movements with the knife towards the dog. Probably over-buoyant with new-found confidence, I tried to be as aggressive as possible. When this torpedo-shaped body of fur, paws and teeth flew through the air at me I made quite a din and lunged forward, slashing away as best I could, given that my resolve was rapidly diminishing to say the least. The beast ignored my knife arm and dug its formidable teeth into my lesser padded arm, shook me to the ground and then began to drag me along. It seemed a while before the handler disengaged him but was actually only a few seconds in reality. No injury was incurred. Once my heart rate subdued and I'd made pals with my four-legged attacker once more, we decided that the session had run its course. I learned never to volunteer again for anything else unless I was absolutely sure what it entailed.

In the mid to late 1960s Her Majesty's Government (HMG) insisted on Civil Defence (CD) training of all police forces lest Great Britain should suffer an atomic bomb attack from a Cold War enemy. In its wisdom HMG was of the opinion that a select group of police officers from throughout England, Wales and Scotland should be trained to protect the public as best they could in order to maintain law and order should such a devastating device be ignited on or over our shores. This manifested itself in the inauguration of Police Mobile Columns (PMC). It was believed that these CD groups would be mobilized and despatched to safer parts of the UK where direct bombing was not anticipated and where bunkers had been prepared for their use. Here they would await a drop in deadly radiation (measured in roentgens) to a safe level, at which point they would emerge and evaluate the situation. I have to say that most of my colleagues who underwent this training were a tad cynical as to it ever working. Some suggested that in reality if an atomic attack was imminent they would do better to grab a bottle or two of whisky (other spirits of choice were obviously available) and make for the nearest nurses' quarters, no doubt to improve their basic first-aid practices required when the lack of roentgens allowed!

One such PMC was set up to test and train the ability of senior Scottish police officers to command under such duress and their subordinate staff to react accordingly and carry out their orders. Officers from several central Scottish police forces were assembled and equipped with army surplus trucks, ambulances, radio-equipped vehicles and mobile kitchens. For a specific exercise the army de-railed an old steam train in unused railway sidings, placing clothed manikin dummies and sound recordings of people groaning in pain or calling out for help in the overturned carriages and underneath piles of coal that had allegedly spilled from the tender of the train when it crashed. It was very realistic.

Several police cadets were chosen to act as casualties and I was one of this lucky band. Shortly before the PMC arrived we were briefed on our role and injuries. I was dressed in a British Rail driver's uniform, then placed with my legs under the coal pile and told to feign unconsciousness but cry out in pain from a severe leg injury if moved. Others were likewise given their roles and placed in and about the overturned carriages. It had been drizzling for some time, but now started in true Scottish fashion to chuck down with rain. The adjudicators dropped by now and then to ensure that we were okay and offer their thanks for our participation. Eventually we were updated on the delay of the PMC which was causing some concerns, coupled with the wet weather. This was due to heavy traffic exiting Glasgow after a Rangers v Celtic football match. I remember exchanging a few comments with fellow participants to the effect that if the PMC hadn't taken into consideration the heavy traffic after a scheduled football match, how on earth were they going to deal with an atomic bomb attack?

When the PMC finally arrived there was a short period while they disembarked from the convoy vehicles and were briefed by their senior officers on their respective tasks. Eventually a group approached the locomotive part of the train, some bearing stretchers and heading to where I lay. Everything was very wet now and some officers who had begun removing coals from the pile around my legs slipped, losing their footing and dropping some of the coals back into the pile. I resolutely maintained my state of unconsciousness (I think). Someone grabbed my body under my arms and attempted to pull me free of the coal, so I let out a loud moan as instructed. Someone else shouted 'Stop, he's injured' so the officer holding me relaxed his grip. I then became aware of a voice whispering in my ear in a gruff Glasgow accent: 'Ye will be f*****g injured son if ye dinnae tell us whit's wrang wi ye.' (In English: 'You will be f******g injured young man if you don't divulge to us the actual nature of the ailment which afflicts you.')

With that I made a quick assessment and informed my saviours that I probably had a compound fracture or broken left ankle. St Andrews ambulance volunteers also involved in this exercise had previously smeared fake blood over this area which was readily visible. Task accomplished, I was finally freed from the coal with some care, strapped onto a stretcher and carried rather haphazardly over the debris from the train and across rough terrain to a military ambulance where the exercise ended as far as me being a casualty was concerned. Glasgow's finest went off to report their actions to their command post and probably grab a much-deserved hot drink and warm themselves up.

The next phase for us cadets was to act as runners between the PMC command posts on site at the train crash and the adjudicator's temporary offices set up nearby, somewhat in the same manner as Lord Baden-Powell used youths that were to become precursors to the Boy Scout movement during the Boer Wars. Coincidentally I'd been patrol leader of Eagle Patrol, 93rd Churchmount Scout Group in Lochgelly for some years previously. As the command post staff made their decisions and formed strategies they would hand us a written version to be taken to the adjudicators. Conversely, the adjudicators supplied us with comments, questions and updates to be delivered to the command posts.

From chats with the various parties I learned that the details of the exercise were that the train had crashed as a result of an act of sabotage while that region of Scotland was on the highest level of alert for a nuclear attack. Apart from the obvious rail disruption and resultant casualties, the train was allegedly carrying a nuclear reactor which may have become unstable; a Scots Guards army officer who was carrying highly secret military correspondence and who was missing; as were two Bengal tigers being shipped between zoos. Highly improbable, you might say, but such is the world of war games.

One such note I took to a command post from the adjudicators I shall never forget. Basically it read that a 999 emergency call had been received from a very frightened bus conductress using a telephone kiosk in the nearby town to the effect that a very large tiger was pacing around encircling the kiosk. State your action. After a few expletives, some chuckles and rolling of eyes, the command team set to laying out their action. While this was going on I took advantage of the mobile kitchen and grabbed a hot drink and a much-needed snack. On my return to the command post the SIO handed me two written responses with express instructions to deliver the one marked 'A' first, await the adjudicator's response, then hand over the one marked 'B'. This I did. Upon opening 'A' the adjudicator burst out laughing and as he handed it around his colleagues they did likewise. I then produced response 'B' which was the official reply and handed it over. While they read this one through, one of the adjudicators showed me note 'A'.

Note 'A', as far as I can recall, claimed that the command post would task an experienced and empathetic officer to phone the bus conductress, offer her relevant advice and tell her not to worry but to remain firmly inside the kiosk. As a matter of urgency a police unit would be despatched with all necessary equipment to deal with this dilemma. The officer asked if she was aware of the only thing that tigers were afraid of. She didn't know, she proclaimed. He then asked if there was a chair inside the kiosk. Again she said no. The officer said that that was a pity because if you'd ever been to a circus then you would have seen the trainer cause the lion or tiger to perform acts while brandishing a chair in front of it. It's a well-known fact therefore that lions and tigers are terrified of chairs. The conversation ended with a reassurance that it wouldn't be long before the police unit, presumably suitably armed with a locally-sourced chair, would be there to free her.

I sincerely hope that all concerned with this response went on to have successful and lengthy careers. It made me laugh for sure. Several years later I attended a concert in London featuring the brilliant Scottish comedian Billy Connolly when he told this same joke with a few alterations. I wonder was this a Billy Connolly original or had he subsequently made it his own?

Nearing the end of my cadetship I was obviously hoping to be appointed constable at the ripe old age of 19 so my final assessment report was very important. As this time approached I received correspondence from Force HQ, Kirkcaldy, informing me that my assessment report was positive and the full contents would be shared with me by my Supt in due course. Furthermore, I'd been selected to attend an Outward Bound course at Fife Constabulary's expense. This was tantamount to saying I would make PC. You can imagine my delight and relief. A six-week arduous physical and mentally stimulating course held in a former military camp just outside the village of Burghead, Morayshire in the north of Scotland lay ahead. What could go wrong? What was there not to like?

Chapter 4

Outward Bound in Burghead on the Moray Firth

After reading through the Outward Bound school itinerary I headed for a local army surplus shop and kitted myself out with what I hoped would be a waterproof anorak (it wasn't), pairs of fleece-lined fatigue trousers, a couple of ex-navy heavy polo-neck jumpers, a pair of stout boots, several pairs of heavy-duty socks, some T-shirts, a pair of mittens, a Russian-style faux fur hat, a sleeping bag and a stout rucksack. The reason for this heavy-duty wardrobe was that my course commenced in February when it's not that clever weather-wise in the village of Burghead on the Moray Firth in the far north-east of Scotland.

The dormitories were spartan but warm and the bunks comfortable. Any problems we thought we might have sleeping would be resolved in a day or two as the physical regime kicked in. Each day started at 0630 hours when a physical training instructor (PTI) shouted us out of our slumber and told us to dress a bit sharpish in our issued plimsolls (gym shoes), gym vest and pants (no socks), and join him on the parade square where he was dressed in a track suit by the way. I'm not saying the plimsolls were flimsy, but rumour had it that if you stood on a coin of the realm you could tell if it was facing heads or tails up. A 3-mile cross-country run then ensued along the beach and back, featuring occasions when we ran up to our knees in really cold sea water. It was February, you may recall. This was followed by a cold shower, a tidy-up of the dormitory in which you were obliged to make your bed 'army fashion' and dress in a manner for whatever was on the daily schedule, then get downstairs for breakfast 'pronto'. Breakfast was actually quite good and plentiful but time was limited so you learned to choose and eat quickly.

The Outward Bound (OB) motto 'To Serve, to Strive, and not to Yield' encompasses the strategy of the founders which, by way of simplification, was 'to unlock a person's full potential through a unique approach to learning and adventure in the wild'. It certainly did that.

There were a handful of other police cadets from Scottish and English forces, three members of the British army junior leader regiment, two guys who were at the end of their Borstal training, the remainder being apprentices from industry and a guy from the equivalent of a public school in Sweden. Not surprisingly, the latter had the best kit of all of us.

We were put through a lot of physical training, both in the gym and on the parade square in full pack order, but we also received a fair amount of class work to teach us survival skills. We had to complete a twenty-four-hour survival test before the next phase of training. The lead PTI was a Kiwi former Royal Marine Commando named Bretell, who we all initially disliked. He had the habit of standing in front of you during lengthy sessions of running on the spot, keeping time by tapping a fencing foil on the ground. The faster he tapped, the faster you ran. Simple and effective. He was very strict and pushed us hard at every physical exercise stage and seemed devoid of humour.

However, as we became fitter, hating him and defying his attempts, as we saw it, to break us, it slowly dawned that what he was trying to accomplish, vis-à-vis improving our fitness and mental agility, was actually for our benefit. He recognized the signs when we were nearly exhausted and would make us rest for a short while. He taught us to rock-climb and abseil, which I'd never done and the thought of it petrified me, as it did a few others. With Bretell's coaxing, support and advice, albeit sometimes harsh, I succeeded in both the ascents and descents sufficiently to continue to the next stage, as did we all. During classes after dinner he and other PTIs explained that the purpose of most of these exercises was to make us realize that our body can endure much more than we think once we reach a state of mind that counteracts the fatigue and pain. They called it 'Going through the pain barrier', or character-building in other words.

The twenty-four-hour survival course found each of us being transported by Jeeps onto a large, bleak moor where we were dropped off individually with instructions to make our way on foot to a map reference, set up an overnight bivouac and then walk to another map reference at a given time the following morning. All we were allowed to carry was a sleeping bag, waterproof poncho, candle, sheath knife, billy-can, eating utensils, can-opener, metal water bottle and a box of matches. To eat we each had a tin of stew, a packet of powdered potatoes (aka pom), a tin of pears, a packet of custard powder, some teabags, a small wrap of sugar and some powdered milk.

After a short hike I chose a likely spot at my given location and using the newly-taught survival skills set to making a lean-to type of shelter with tree branches and bracken. I collected twigs, branches and pine cones as the makings of a fire. We'd been told to drink a hot drink often to combat the cold. It was damn cold too. After dark I set the fire and started my evening meal. The candle wouldn't stay in because of the wind and I needed to preserve matches so packed up trying. In relative darkness I started heating the stew and thought, what the hell, I'll just add the pom and stir it all in. When done I tucked in with gusto, only to find that the pom I'd added was in fact the custard powder. Had I invented a recipe for a sort of sweet and sour stew? I was cold, hungry and tired so I ate it, followed by pears for dessert. It wasn't too bad actually.

I slept sparingly in my sleeping bag with the poncho over my head, then after a pom and tea brekkie dismantled my bivouac and hiked off towards the pick-up point. En route I saw one or two of my colleagues walking in the same direction as myself from various parts of the moor. When we met up it seemed that we'd all been dropped off within a mile or so of one another but not within sight due to the rough terrain. Still, we'd all survived, some better than others. Surprisingly, one of the army junior leader guys couldn't hack the dark so he just huddled down in a dry ditch near his designated map reference and waited the night out. The PTIs who picked us up in the minibus had a couple of flasks of hot sweet tea with them; they made sure he had the lion's share of that.

Back at the OB school we had a large, hot and very welcome lunch, then a not-so-welcome cold shower followed by an interesting and relaxed debrief during which we learned that the next phase of our course was to be a four-day hike and bivouac above the snow line in Glen Affric. A fantastic opportunity to further test our skills, fitness and leadership qualities. It was going to be one hell of a challenge. Bring it on!

Meanwhile we were undergoing seamanship training on a fine three-masted yacht which the OB owned. Rowing seven-man cutters regularly out of the harbour was heavy going but necessary as we needed to be competent in their use before we set sail for a few days negotiating the fabulous Scandinavian fjords. We successfully completed 'man overboard' drills which were very tricky as the temperature in the sea at that point and time of the year was pretty damn cold. We'd drawn straws to be the 'casualty' which was won, or some pessimists said lost, by one of the army guys. We rowed just outside the harbour wall, then he slid over the side and we rowed away and took a circular route to return and save him. This took several minutes and as the waves rebounded off the breakwater the casualty started shouting at us. A few of his south London-accented expletives advised us to get a bloody move on. When we pulled him into the boat only a few minutes later his teeth were chattering with cold and he shivered violently so he was wrapped in a blanket and given some hot sweet tea from the ubiquitous PTIs' flasks. Hot sweet tea was undeniably the fix-all here, it seemed. It did the trick for him then and others at different times during our various exercises and tests.

As we reached the end of the course and reflected on all of the major trials and varied challenges that had come our way and that we had successfully overcome, virtually to a man we now worshipped the very ground that Bretell walked on. He and his team had made sure that we did, in fact, serve, strive and did not yield. Well done them and, of course, us!

There's no doubt in my mind that the OB experience made me a better and more balanced person. I matured and learned, not only from the instructors but from the varied lives and comradeship of fellow students on my course, including the lads from Borstal training. It goes without saying that I never felt fitter. There were many occasions in later life when I reflected on this course and drew strength from the many and varied lessons learned there. I am most grateful to the Outward Bound Trust, as it's now known, for all it gave me and more especially to Fife Constabulary for sending and funding me through it. I would recommend the OBT to any young person seeking to improve themselves.

Chapter 5

Fife Constabulary's First PC 600

Until I was sworn in as a police constable there had only ever been a total of 598 PCs in Fife Constabulary at one time. The six of us that were enrolled that day in April 1967 took the number up to 604. My shoulder number was 600. The very first. I was pretty damn chuffed. Was this an omen of things to come?

Like all other PCs before us, we attended Tulliallan Castle, the Scottish Police Training College. It was, and still is, a fine police college and I thoroughly enjoyed learning Scottish criminal law and police procedures there. Probationer PCs from many Scottish police forces were part of my intake. Apart from the classroom sessions, reading up on law and police procedures accompanied by relevant lectures, our instructors taught us how to deal with rudimentary situations such as attending a domestic dispute; action to be taken upon arrival at the scene of a motor vehicle accident; powers of Stop and Search; basic arrest procedures and giving evidence in court; all through practical exercises. Regular physical exercise in the gym, cross-country runs and swimming involving personal survival training in the college pool were mandatory, as was first-aid training, for obvious reasons. There was also an emphasis on marching drills which were meant to instil self-discipline, pride in the uniform and teach us teamwork and positive response to instructions.

After sixteen weeks of intensive training we were all immensely proud to hear the order barked out by the senior drill instructor at the end of a lengthy march past and display of manual traffic direction signals for us to march off the parade square to the tune of *Blue Bonnets over the Border* played by a fine Scottish police pipe band. We'd passed out (as in graduated, not fainted). We'd successfully passed all tests and challenges placed before us and were now to return to our respective police forces to be fine-tuned in local legislation and procedures before being unleashed upon the unsuspecting public.

Post-Tulliallan, we probationary Fife PCs were temporarily based at HQ Kirkcaldy to learn more about local county byelaws and Fife Constabulary procedures. During this period there was an outbreak of the deadly virus epizootic lymphangitis in a farm nearby so a couple of us 'rookies' were despatched to assist local officers dealing with same along with the Ministry of Agriculture and Fisheries personnel on site. Epizootic lymphangitis is a highly contagious disease found mainly in horses and caused by the fungus histoplasma farciminosum. Cattle and humans can be affected, but thankfully this is rare. Chickens are also susceptible, however. If not contained there's a danger of the virus spreading and epidemic status being reached. As with anthrax in cattle, culling would ensue. After being issued with wellies, rubber gloves and face masks, we rookies were briefed by the on-site Ministry officials and shown how to operate a stirrup pump. With this we sprayed disinfectant over the tyres of every motor vehicle entering or leaving the farm as well as ensuring that all pedestrian visitors stepped through a shallow metal tray containing a strong disinfectant. Undeniably a most important but thoroughly boring task. Was this what all my recent police training was about?

After a couple of weeks at HQ I was assigned to Methil Police Station. Methil was then a small industrial port that served the local distillery and paper manufacturing works as well as the coal-mining industry. There was still a small fishing fleet. A large bonded warehouse was situated in the dock area. Deep sea fishing flourished and foreign merchant ships frequented the docks, bringing their cargos and crews from afar. The town, however, was suffering from the gradual demise of the coal industry and unemployment was rife, therefore petty crime flourished. Shops and small businesses were closing down with alarming regularity. Methil is also the home ground of East Fife Football Club at Bayview Park. East Fife was then one of several of Fife's lesser-known football clubs but very important to the sport as a training ground for local talent. Is there such a thing as local football talent these days?

Due to the presence of the bonded warehouse and the fact that the docks had been part of the Royal Naval dockyard at Rosyth, a few miles west along the coast, during the Second World War it had been protected by Ministry of Defence police for many years. According to several of my longer-serving peers, when Fife Constabulary took responsibility for this role the facility of 'indulgence' persisted. This was similar to the issue of a tot of rum in the Royal Navy. If the temperature dropped to a given level, usually during night duty in winter, then PCs assigned to the dock beat would be met at a pre-arranged time and place on their rounds by a duty sergeant who would dispense the indulgence against their signature in his pocketbook. Apparently one of these sergeants also took a sip of rum himself at these times. Sadly it was not available by the time I was assigned to Methil.

This reminds me of another tale passed on to me during a quiet night duty by a colleague who had served in the navy. One of the Royal Navy's ageing aircraft carriers was on a decommissioning tour of former Commonwealth countries before she was due to be broken up on return to the UK. A few days' sail away from Egypt a member of the crew contacted the Queen Alexandra's Royal Army Nursing Corps based in that country, inviting them to a soirée when the ship docked there. The nurses gladly accepted the invitation, so shortly before they were due to arrive a galvanized basin was obtained, bedecked in crepe paper and set up to hold a liquid punch to be offered to the guests as they boarded. Several recipes were considered and tried but one of the Chief Petty Officers (CPOs), who designated himself as the official taster, thought they were too weak. He added a drop or two of several spirits, then a drop or two, maybe three, of some others and, when happy with the result, instructed those deployed to ensure that each guest was offered a glass as she alighted the gangplank and was piped aboard in traditional naval fashion. This was duly done. A little while after festivities had begun, one of these junior ratings approached the CPO and asked him to accompany him to the punch bowl where he pointed out that the galvanized area on the inside of the bowl below the crepe paper was 'bubbling'. Closer examination revealed that the galvanization was being eroded, presumably by the alcohol in the punch. Needless to say, the remaining contents were swiftly disposed of. Whether any of the guests had any problematic symptoms as a result of consuming this questionable beverage was not disclosed to me, or the guests either presumably. One can only guess. Hopefully a good time was had by all.

This same colleague was also proud to divulge that over some considerable period of time the engine-room crew on this massive craft had examined in great detail the several miles of piping and identified the down drainage pipe into which the remains of the daily issue of rum (tot) was poured after the ceremony ceased. It was customary for the

OIC (Officer in Charge) of the tot issue to receive same from a CPO who scooped the measure out of a rum barrel, broken open daily for this use, into a small metal cup and handed it to each rating for consumption. Any leftovers were tipped down a drain. Certain CPOs would insert their thumb surreptitiously into the tot measure ladle, thus displacing a small amount per issue. By the end of the issue this amounted to a fair amount of rum. The CPO would then ring from the deck at the end of the ceremony and alert the engine-room crew that the dregs were on their way. The engine-room crew had fitted a tap at the end of a small pipe they had inserted into this particular pipe and would simply turn it to open and so catch the rum residue in a receptacle. This 'bonus' was shared between the engine crew and CPOs in on the act later in the day. Naval ingenuity at its best, obviously.

As a bachelor I was supplied with a list of addresses where local and screened landladies provided rooms for rent to single police officers. Most were widows and some police widows. I chose a lovely lady named Mrs Kinnear who kept an immaculate semi-detached property in a good part of town. She already provided lodgings for another officer at Methil police station so she was obviously a good prospect. Mrs Kinnear had run a popular small café/restaurant with her husband which she gave up upon his demise. One of her two sons still lived at home. He was paraplegic so wasn't able to find full-time employment and was well-known and a popular figure around town. Over the ensuing months I came to enjoy his company and Mrs Kinnear's cooking was fantastic. She became like a second mum to me. Her dictum that if any of her lodgers entertained a lady friend in their room they had to leave the door open was particularly appreciated by my proper mother.

Mrs Kinnear still kept in touch with individuals who had supplied her with fresh produce when she ran the local café with her hubby. Some of these 'suppliers' would appear at the rear door of her property late in the evening and after a quiet discourse she'd place the produce, often wrapped in newspaper, in a chest freezer in the scullery. It didn't take a Sherlock to realize that some of these items had been obtained by poaching from the large country estates that were to be found all around this region of Fife. Poaching, although illegal, was commonly accepted by the local population, especially those on low incomes. During my time in residence there many brown trout, several fine salmon and the occasional side of venison came into the Kinnear household in this way. I felt it prudent not to embarrass this fine lady with any questions concerning her purchases and the source of same, but implied I wasn't happy with such transactions as it could reflect poorly on my profession and may affect her reputation as well. I know she simply ignored my advice. It is, of course, a fact that I enjoyed the tasty and nutritious meals that she provided using these grand ingredients.

After such a venison delivery Mrs Kinnear concocted a tasty venison soup, venison sausages, mince and tatties – naturally incorporating venison mince – venison cold cuts and venison steaks for our delectation almost daily for about a fortnight. During a night duty meal break around this time I opened my lunchbox and produced a sandwich which contained – you've guessed it – more bloody venison! I blurted out 'Not bloody venison again', much to the surprise and consternation of my older and married colleagues, some of whom I think thought me a spoiled brat at that moment. After explaining that my outburst was brought about by the abundance of venison in my diet of late, I swapped sandwiches and I think relished a Kraft cheese slice and tomato one for my sins.

It was Mrs K's habit to have a night off on a Thursday evening when she would play bingo with some female friends in a local hall. On those evenings she would prepare a salad dinner for us that was left in the fridge. She was of that generation of women who believed that men couldn't be trusted to cook for themselves, bless her. On one such occasion I was on night duty. It was winter and a fair amount of snow fell, not helped by strong winds. I was on a foot beat and at about 2.00 am noticed the blue lamp flashing on top of one of our police/public call boxes. I picked up the receiver, only to be told by the desk sergeant to make my way back to the station as soon as possible. I asked why but he just said: 'Soon as ye can lad.' Walking briskly was tricky given the snow and wind, but after about half an hour I made it. The sergeant was grinning when he told me that I had a visitor in the inspector's office. When I went in, there was Mrs Kinnear. I asked what was wrong, to which she replied: 'Nothing, but as you hadn't had a proper dinner I didn't want you to be cold or hungry so I brought you some hot soup.' She then produced a thermos flask. She'd walked a couple of miles in the snow in the wee small hours to deliver it to me. I was so embarrassed. After thanking her, I arranged her a lift home with the aid of said sergeant. You can imagine the mickey-taking I received from my peers.

I policed areas where many coal mines were located and I used to visit them for a number of official and sometimes unofficial reasons. I've always had great respect for the hardy individuals who worked the coal, suffered the hardships of mining and the resultant hazards of debilitating respiratory disease that is symptomatic of that industry. I recall only too well the grey and sad-looking faces of many of these men who obviously had too little sun and too little fresh air, whose bodies were wracked with fearful bouts of coughing or bent over with acute arthritis, as was the case with one of my uncles. On the few occasions I had to visit the local GP, the waiting room was nearly always filled with such men. Their attempts to breathe and chest-rattling coughs were testimony to what mining had so unfairly extracted from them and an indication that they would probably not make old bones.

I was thankful that I was not to be part of this working lifestyle. Even had I wanted to, it was blatantly obvious that any future in coal-mining would be short-lived as collieries were regularly closing down all around. I had Di mainly to thank for that. He urged me to work hard at my studies at Beath High School and told me that if he could advise me on only one subject, it was not to enter the coal industry; advice which I readily took, I'm happy to say. On the whole the miners were a decent, hard-working bunch, honest and surprisingly cheerful given their awful working conditions, relatively poor lifestyle and often substandard accommodation.

I regularly popped in for a cuppa in the canteens while on patrol and talked among the miners about football or local events that affected them. Being from a family of miners was obviously an advantage. Even as a young recruit it gave me an opportunity to gain their trust as their local bobby. Some who knew my Di and my uncles had apparently given me their vote of confidence and let their peers know that I was okay and could be trusted. This was essential for me to be able to successfully work among them and represent law and order in their towns, especially the public houses, although it was sometimes difficult to obtain and in fact maintain.

As a football fan I quite enjoyed being assigned to the odd match at Bayview Park. Although not an East Fife supporter, I enjoyed that percentage of the match that was available for us to watch, given that we were supposed to be patrolling and keeping the Queen's peace. For a normal game there was a complement of a sergeant and four or five PCs in the ground and a van crew outside. The sergeant normally stayed in an office over the stand so he had an overview of the pitch. On a good day attendance would be in the hundreds, so not a large public order event. We PCs patrolled the cindered perimeter of the playing area in pairs and at a relatively slow pace. There were no stewards in those days. At half-time we tucked into a mug of hot Bovril and a mutton pie, which were especially welcome in the winter months. The east wind that blew up the steep hill from the docks coming off the North Sea was brutally cold at times.

East Fife drew top-of-the-league Glasgow Rangers in a Scottish football cup round. Rangers would bring a horde of supporters and not all of them would be law-abiding. A special unit of Glasgow City Police always accompanied these supporters to away games so that would be a great help as they could identify any troublemakers. On the day an inspector, two sergeants and, as far as my memory will permit, eight to ten PCs were assigned to the ground. During the pre-match briefing the inspector, an avuncular and pleasant chap, suggested to the PCs assigned to patrolling and crowd control duties within the stadium: 'Walk much faster around the pitch so that the supporters will think there are more of you.' I nearly laughed out loud. Was that the strategy? My suggestion that we would need to cover up our shoulder numbers in that case was met with some derision by one of the sergeants, adding 'Typical know-all ex-cadet.' I was only trying to help. The match went without incident thankfully, mainly because Rangers won comfortably. I noticed that I wasn't selected for football duty for a couple of games afterwards. Probably coincidence.

Chapter 6

Dealing with my First Dead Body

I think I'd been a PC for just over a year before I dealt with my first dead body. This was in 1968 when I reached the ripe old age of 20 and the year Dunfermline Athletic Football Club (the Pars), then managed by the late legendary Jock Stein, won the Scottish Cup for the first and probably only time. Not well-known outside of Scotland, mainly because of the deserved celebrations conducted over another soccer game played at Wembley Stadium a couple of years earlier when a talented England side defeated their arch-enemy Germany and quite rightly lifted the Jules Rimet Trophy (World Cup) for, so far at least, the only time. Incidentally, an aspiring talented young footballer by the name of Alex Ferguson was playing for the Pars then. He went on to do well as the manager of Aberdeen Football Club and extremely well as the manager of arguably the world's best-supported and finest football team, namely Manchester United. The same late great Jock Stein went on to successfully manage the mighty Glasgow Celtic FC and then Scotland's national team to success far and beyond their capabilities for a small nation playing on a world platform. To pinch a line from Scotland's unofficial national sporting anthem, 'When shall we see his like again?'

I remember that the unfortunate deceased was a small, elderly female, whose bloated and lifeless body was spotted one evening floating in the cold, dark grey waters in the harbour of a Fife seaside village near East Wemyss. I later found out at the post mortem that she'd been in the sea for some time. It seems that she'd entered the sea somewhere near Newcastle accidentally or may have committed suicide; we never did determine which. It is not uncommon for the sea currents around the East Neuk of Fife to occasionally deposit dead bodies on those shores after they've entered the sea further down the Scottish east coast or even from English waters.

Another PC and I commandeered a small row boat and rowed out to where she'd been spotted by a harbour worker and, with as much dignity as we could muster, retrieved her small but heavy body into the dinghy, placing it into a coffin-shaped shell we'd taken out for the purpose. Once we transferred her to the local mortuary my colleague left me alone to prepare her for the inevitable post-mortem examination which was to be carried out on behalf of the PF the next day. The PF (Procurator Fiscal), more frequently referred to as the Fiscal, is the locally-appointed legal representative to whom the police report sudden or suspicious deaths such as these. The Fiscal decides whether the circumstances of such incidents warrant further investigation or closes the enquiry and instructs the police to notify the next of kin accordingly in order for them to arrange the return of the body of their loved one into their charge. This is necessary in order to establish the cause of death and hopefully the identity of the person as well as ensuring that if the cause of death was not occasioned naturally, a criminal investigation would be initiated forthwith.

It was also customary police practice, but not actual force policy, that the newest recruited officer carried out this function by way of learning the trade. In reality it was also a way in which more experienced officers who disliked dealing with dead bodies could avoid doing so. While searching the lady's clothing in the morgue looking for any obvious evidence as to her identity, I discovered she was wearing an old blue canvas Royal Navy issue money belt under her corsetry. In this were some personal identity documents plus £80 cash in used sterling English banknotes. Also present, inexplicably, was a sodden bag of mint sweets; such an unusual place to keep one's sweets. After logging the property in my issue pocketbook and while preparing a typed report for the pathologist and ultimately the PF's office, I looked over her body to see if there were any obvious marks of violence or anything at all unusual. I saw nothing other than the expected cadaver disruption caused by her immersion in water for a lengthy period, during which she had become a food source for crustaceans and the like. When I later told my colleagues about this back at the police station, many agreed that they didn't take kindly to this line of work. Some of them admitted that they couldn't do it. I'd found out that I could, and surprisingly I found it extremely interesting trying to figure out who she was, et cetera:

- Where had she come from?
- How had she come to be in the sea?
- How long had she been there?

These were some of the unknown facts that were fascinating and intriguing to me:

- What had this lady been like in life?
- Was she someone's mother, sister or loved one?
- Had she left children behind?
- Was she missed and had someone reported her as a missing person?

Little did I know then that this was to be the start of a trend that would grimly but rightly follow me throughout my career and carry on into my endeavours after retirement from the police service. Ironically this incident, my first brush with dealing with death, was to cause me a bit of a problem and no little cause for reappraisal of my chosen career in the not-too-distant months, of which more later.

As I progressed through the trials and tribulations of the obligatory two years of a PC's training known as the probationary period, learning to deal with drunks, common assaults, minor traffic violations and petty thefts, I yearned to become a detective. I didn't want to just spend my time, as I saw it then, as a glorified watchman 'shaking hands with padlocks' on night duty and directing traffic on day shift. I wanted to investigate more challenging crimes and make a difference to victims by apprehending those responsible for violations against them and hopefully tracing and returning their stolen property. A short attachment to the CID had whetted my appetite in this regard. I was aware that I'd received a favourable report while engaged with the CID and I knew that I could prove myself in this field if given the chance.

The practice of dealing with property in a rural Fife Constabulary police station at that time was to store any small sums of money in a property store in the station within a signed and sealed envelope until it was required to be returned to the rightful owner or their representative. A record of this was made in the officer's pocketbook as well as any relevant police report. Any larger sums were entered accordingly and kept in the station inspector's safe. This was the procedure I carried out with the elderly lady's cash. After listing the serial number of each banknote in my pocketbook, which was then checked and signed by the duty sergeant at the time of entry, I placed it in my personal locker with the intention of transferring it to the inspector's safe when we were both next on duty. In reality we often stuck such items in our personal lockers for temporary safekeeping and then transferred them to the property store at a later time when less busy. This had been my intention, but I simply forgot about it. Also the thought of anyone employed at the station stealing it never entered my head. A sharp lesson I was soon to learn at some cost.

Six months or so later after the PF's enquiry determined that this lady's tragic death was accidental I was instructed to forward the money and personal correspondence to HQ in order for it to be restored to a relative. When I checked my locker, the envelope was missing. I couldn't believe it. I hadn't noticed it or even thought about it for several months because of all the stuff I'd gathered and kept there. My locker, like those of many other colleagues, was chock full of winter and lightweight uniform items, sports kit, civilian clothes and the bric-a-brac generally kept by all officers in these rather compact metal receptacles. After exhausting my search with the aid of a few colleagues, I eventually had to go cap-in-hand to a sergeant and formally report my dilemma. This was tantamount to an admission of neglect of duty and the first time I had lost or misplaced anything important in my career.

The sergeant conducted his own search of my locker, the room space generally around and under it as well as those of neighbouring officers, but unfortunately to no good effect. He then was obliged to formally report the loss to Divisional HQ at Kirkcaldy. I filled out a detailed report outlining the circumstances of the loss while feeling rather embarrassed. Several days later when I reported for duty I was summoned to the inspector's office and introduced to a Detective Inspector (DI) and Detective Constable (DC) from HQ CID.

Chapter 7

Accused of Theft

They wasted no time in asking me if I'd taken the money. I told them emphatically that I had not. I was appalled that they would even consider this possibility, but after all I was young in service and somewhat naïve regarding internal police investigations. My pride was hurt that they could even think this of me, a fellow police officer. However, they were obviously quite correct in considering that I could have taken it and quite right to interview me as a suspect.

Ironically, just a few weeks before this loss was discovered I had purchased a used Mini motor car from a local garage where it had been rebuilt after being involved in a serious accident. Apart from being a garish canary yellow colour, it was very cheap. This was by way of part-exchanging an even older Ford Prefect I'd purchased from a local midwife solely to learn to drive and in which I'd successfully passed my driving test. Plus, would you believe, the princely sum of £80 cash. This was a combination of money I'd saved and a small loan from my mother. A dog handler attached to the police station had apparently made the investigators aware of this purchase. It had taken these officers no time at all to incorrectly decide that the cash I had paid for the Mini and the money I reported lost were one and the same.

During the interrogation, for that was what it felt like, they told me that this looked bad for me. Even with my limited police experience, I knew how little impact this fact would really have. It was only circumstantial, after all. They went on to say that unless I saw sense and admitted my guilt, they would interview the garage owner who had sold me the car. They would have to speak to my mother who had allegedly loaned me some of the money, and make enquiries of my friends, associates and local business people to ensure, or otherwise, my honesty, integrity and financial standing. Copies of my bank account would also be requested and scrutinized. Standard investigative procedure, I thought, none of which would infer my guilt or innocence for that matter.

When I reiterated my innocence the DI told me that he didn't believe me and then much to my surprise he formally cautioned me and had me placed in a cell. I was required to remove my belt, tie and bootlaces and then the door was slammed shut; the very same cell door I had closed on people I'd arrested time and time again. It was surreal. I was devastated. This could not be happening to me. It was obviously a ploy by the investigators to let me sweat it out and induce me to admit to the crime; a crime I had not committed. At the very most I was guilty of being a bit negligent, but in my opinion that didn't merit being 'banged up'. After all, making mistakes is a part of any learning experience.

My beloved Di, the most important male influence in my life, coupled with my mother, had instilled a sound sense of honesty in me and urged me to tell the truth from a very young age. His father had been a police officer in a small and now defunct local constabulary and he had been strictly brought up to always respect others and their property. I knew my mum's life would be shattered too because she was so proud of my achievements thus far. I was well aware that the detectives would make play of the fact that being my mother, she would therefore say she had loaned me the money even if she hadn't, blood being thicker than water and all that. Clearly they did not know my mother and her complete sense of honesty.

If I'd lied about my mother lending me the cash I used to purchase the car she would not have backed me up and would have told them so. She would not lie for me. Apart from being entirely honest, she was also quite religious. I didn't want her to have to go through any unnecessary trauma, but couldn't see any way out. She'd have to know what I'd been accused of and we'd both have to deal with any repercussions. Overriding all of this was the simple fact that I had not taken or used the money in any way.

An embarrassed fellow officer eventually brought me a mug of tea and something to read and told me that I was not to be engaged in conversation or receive visitors but to be treated as 'incommunicado'. To say the least I was beginning to think the worst when an extremely popular sergeant stationed at Methil opened the cell door and 'sprang me'. I was never so pleased to see the larger-than-life Sergeant Jim McNeill, believe me. He was the father of one of my closest friends (also named Jim), who'd similarly been a Fife police cadet and is now a retired Met police officer like myself.

He took me to his office, sat me down and cut to the quick. Had I taken the money, he demanded? No, I told him, and he knew I meant it. 'In that case you've got nothing to worry about son,' said he. I tried hard to believe him. He telephoned HQ and told a member of the CID that I was now in his custody and I would be remaining in my lodgings until they wanted to interview me again. He insisted that at such time he would be present to ensure my rights were accorded me, as my 'friend' to use police parlance. The term 'friend' in such cases denotes an officer of higher rank than the officer being interviewed in disciplinary or internal affairs matters, or quite simply my legal representative, who would advise me of my rights and ensure that I was treated fairly and correctly and not made to feel vulnerable, intimidated or bullied by a senior investigating officer. After all, police officers are entitled to be deemed innocent until proven guilty in the same way as any other member of our civilized society, although certain elements in that society would like to see this right rescinded.

Several days later this interview took place in Sergeant McNeill's office. The DI simply started by stating that the Chief Constable had empowered him to state that I would be allowed to resign if I admitted taking the money because it was not in the public interest to prosecute me. Whether this was true or not I'm still not sure, nor probably ever will be. I suspect it was subterfuge. I told him, for the umpteenth time, that I had not taken the money. Would I have listed the notes, their denominations and actual serial numbers in my pocketbook which was then checked and signed by my supervising sergeant when, while alone in the mortuary, I could simply have pocketed them without anyone knowing? I don't think so. This remark seemed to irritate him because he then said: 'So you thought about it then?'

The interview, for this was milder in attitude than the first time he'd questioned me, abruptly terminated. I was released uncharged and after a few days idling away in my digs a colleague popped in to tell me to report for duty as usual the following morning while HQ decided what course of action, if any, should be taken. I was advised to put this matter to the back of my mind and get on with my work. Easier said than done, believe me. Even the lovely Mrs Kinnear thought I'd been dealt with poorly.

Not long afterwards I appeared before the inspector at my local police station. It was all a bit formal as he read out the report from HQ CID as I stood at ease before his desk, hands clasped behind my back with my uniform cap held under my left armpit in the accepted manner. At the conclusion of this procedure he told me to take a seat, then gave me advice on how to deal better with property in my charge and officially reprimanded me for losing the money and failing to properly secure it in his safe. He then informed me that no further action was to be taken and I should put the experience behind me, learn from it, and get on with my career. This I did, but with an altered vision of life generally and more especially with regard to my chosen career path. Ironically it made me more determined to join the CID because I was of the considered opinion that even with my then limited interview experience I could have carried out a better investigation than that of the hapless DI and DC from HQ.

Chapter 8

Disillusioned of Fife

I began to become somewhat disillusioned with my lot with what I now viewed as antiquated policing methods and the culture of doing things the way they had always been done instead of looking for ways to improve procedures. I began to look outwardly towards other larger police forces if I should decide to remain within the police. I researched the Royal Canadian Mounted Police (RCMP) and London's Metropolitan Police (Met) as well as the RAF Police as possibilities, so I wrote to them seeking the possibility of a position and/or transfer. The travel bug was beginning to bite and I sought new challenges.

I was working a stretch of 6.00 pm to 2.00 am night duties in order to assist rural officers during their busier holiday periods. This part of East Fife regularly attracts a great many tourists, especially holidaymakers from the Glasgow area during the summer months known as the Glasgow Fair and many villages put on special events to encourage tourism. Needless to say, the occasional spot of bother occurs and the home beat officers need assistance. Many of these rural officers worked in small villages on their own, known as single stations, and needed help particularly at pub closing times but also with other enquiries when corroboration was required in order to comply with Scottish law and deal with any legal questions raised in future court proceedings. Often this assistance was also provided by well-minded locals who enlisted in the Special Constabulary.

PC Ian Campbell, the husband of my favourite cousin, was one of these experienced rural constables so I knew how much and why these single station officers needed assistance as a result of the many chats we'd had together prior to me entering the police service and since I'd done so. A great deal of the responsibility for my ever having become a police officer must lie at his door. He was a very good role model for me, not only then as a young impressionable constable seeking professional help and advice but also, and maybe more importantly, as a very decent human being, husband and father. I learned a great deal from him and my cousin Irene and I'm extremely proud of their support, love and companionship throughout my career.

Around this time it was customary for a particular soon-to-retire sergeant to hold a card school by way of relaxation during the night duty meal break which occasionally went on a little longer than the allotted forty-five minutes if things were quiet. His fellow players were generally long-serving PCs who were mostly ex-servicemen like himself. On a particularly wet and windy winter's night I walked into the police station just before 2.00 am to book off duty and asked if there was any chance of a lift to my lodgings. This request was dismissed out of hand by the sergeant so I pulled my civvy raincoat over my uniform and headed off on foot for the 2-mile walk. What the hell. I was young and fit and could do with the exercise, I told myself while actually cursing him under my breath as I walked home in the bleak, cold night with the wind and rain piercing my coat and stinging my face.

As I trudged along the dank, dark streets and alleyways, my body bent into the sleeting rain, I saw a couple of figures moving about in the car park outside Bayview Park, the town's then second division football club ground. They obviously hadn't seen me so I huddled into a shop doorway and kept watch. I had no personal radio, so calling for assistance was not an option. There was no public phone kiosk visible. As I observed my quarry I saw and heard one of them smash what I later discovered to be the quarter light, in the days when most cars had them, on the driver's side window, then watched as he pulled back into the shadows, presumably to wait and see if anyone had heard. They both walked back to the car, looked around, then opened the driver's door and climbed in. I recognized it as an old model Ford Prefect because I'd owned one prior to buying the accursed yellow Mini.

I ran towards them still unseen and heard the engine burst into life literally as I drew alongside. I'd drawn my truncheon and held my handcuffs ready for use. This was a rough area and I knew better than to simply approach two males and politely ask what they were up to, even as a police officer. I swiftly and rather deftly, although I say so myself, snapped one end of the cuffs around a wrist of the youth in the driver's seat, the other end I locked around the steering wheel. His head was bent below the dashboard where he'd been hot-wiring the car's ignition system so he was a bit surprised. He'd obviously neither seen nor heard my approach. The other youth was rummaging through the rear seats so I reached in and grabbed him. I think the sight of the truncheon spoke for itself because he didn't put up a struggle and I soon held him in a restraint position. What to do now? I didn't have my personal radio and no-one else was around to assist me. Here I was, technically off-duty with two prisoners in my custody, one or both of whom could easily cut up rough when they realized I was on my own. Only one thing to do, I thought. Use my initiative.

If the mountain couldn't come to Mohammed, then Mohammed must go to the mountain as the saying goes. After cautioning and formally arresting them for attempting to take and drive away a motor vehicle, I handcuffed them to one another and placed them in the rear of the two-door car. After warning them not to do anything daft, I drove the short distance to the police station. If anyone had been watching it must have looked like a scene straight out of *Dixon of Dock Green* which was a very popular London-based police TV series of the time.

Pleased with myself for my off-duty apprehensions, I locked the police yard gates once we arrived at the station and marched the youths from the back of the stolen car into the rear entrance of the station. I was not totally surprised to find some of the night-duty staff sitting around the muster room table still engaged in a card game with the almost-retired sergeant acting as dealer. They looked up in surprise at my entrance as I took the youths through to the cells where I searched them, placing one of them in a detention room and the other in a cell to avoid collusion.

After completing this task, I was heading back out to the yard to search the vehicle when the sergeant asked me what I was doing. When I told him the facts he looked at me rather incredulously and then followed me out while I checked out the Ford Prefect. By now I was coming to the realization that the sergeant was not over-enamoured by my untimely intrusion. When I'd finished searching the car he beckoned me to his office, probably not for a meritorious award, I remember thinking. How right I was. He despatched the card-players to their various posts, which didn't seem to please them either. When that was done he asked me again to go through my actions in detail. After I'd finished speaking he sat silently for a while obviously deep in thought with his fingers forming the shape of a steeple under his chin apparently chewing over my evidence, or lack of it as I was beginning to wonder. What then followed totally surprised and then angered me, and ultimately made my mind up that it was now time for a change of venue, if not profession.

After briefly praising my swift thinking and innovative arrests, not to mention my courage, he berated me for making him and the rest of the night duty look like they were not doing their job. This was pretty rich coming from a guy who was engaged in a card game throughout the affair and blatantly not properly attending to his constabulary duties. I argued that even if all of the PCs had been on their beats or patrols it didn't mean that they would have seen what I'd seen; after all, I had simply walked into the incident on my way home. He ignored this sensible plea and continued in the vein of me making him look less than professional. Then he dropped the bombshell. The upshot was, as he saw it, I had aided and abetted the theft of a motor vehicle. What he meant to say, I think, was that I'd driven the car as an uninsured person. Because I was only trained as a GP (General Purpose) police driver at that time, which is the basic standard, I should not have driven the car. Technically I was not authorized or insured by the constabulary for this purpose. That said, under the circumstances other factors had taken over in my opinion and I simply overlooked this technicality. I had no means of communication to summon assistance and I didn't fancy escorting my prisoners back to the nick on foot. I argued that if the worst came to the worst I'd probably only get a reprimand from a senior officer, a sort of smack on the back of the hand because the arrests would hopefully take priority. Was the owner going to sue me or the constabulary for driving his car without his permission under the circumstances? His real reasoning was still self-preservation, methinks.

I was instructed to complete my notes and leave all of the outstanding enquiries to him. The owner would be informed and asked to collect his car after making a written statement as to any damage caused, etc. Meanwhile, the CID would deal with the prisoners in the morning. In other words his night-duty shift would get recognition for a good job well done and the CID would endeavour to obtain admissions of other crimes from the two miscreants. I was to be satisfied with literally a pat on the head because as I was only a rookie I didn't fully understand the way things were. On the contrary, I knew well what it was all about. He knew I was not going to upset the apple cart. One didn't then. I should accept his advice and that was that. Everyone would benefit from this situation. No-one would appear to be other than efficient and true professionals getting on with their job. Even more disillusioned now, I walked slowly and pensively home, all the while contemplating my immediate future.

I could not and would not continue to operate in such a small-minded environment. The majority of my colleagues were hard-working and honest professionals. Good people to be around. Sincere in their efforts to help the society in which they lived and worked. Yet a very small minority, like this chevron-bedecked dinosaur, were uniform-carriers. In other words they wanted all of the benefits of wearing the uniform but did little actual work to deserve to be part of the very proud tradition of a police service which was, and still is, envied throughout the world. I should know because I went on to work on criminal investigations in many countries as you will read about later.

It will come as no surprise to the reader that the following evening when I reported for duty I learned that I had actually been quite a small part of the previous evening's arrests scenario. The apprehensions had basically only come to fruition due to the experienced direction of a certain sergeant and his shift PCs had reacted accordingly. The CID had extracted a number of admissions to other car thefts and local burglaries from these two young thieves, resulting in the recovery of stolen goods in other local petty criminals' addresses which brought about more arrests. This was not the way it was supposed to be, according to staff at the Scottish Police Training School which I'd attended for many rigorous weeks at Tulliallan Castle but it was the way of the real world as I was learning. At least I'd been given a mention and not ruled out altogether.

It is fair to say that my time with Fife Constabulary was mostly very happy and informative and I learned a great deal about policing which was to stand me in good stead throughout my career. I met a few special people who have remained life-long friends for which I shall always be truly thankful. There were many great and interesting characters. One that springs to mind was a sergeant who took me under his wing and taught me many of the real aspects of the job. Not the ones churned out by the training staff who mostly preferred any sedentary position to actually walking the streets wearing the blue and dealing with the Great British public face-to-face rather than via a training manual. He had, however, a funny little flaw, or rather an eccentricity, in as much as he often attempted to extend his diction in excess of his vocabulary, often using the wrong words in the wrong place. Still, none of us is perfect (or is it prefect), as anyone who knows me well could confirm. I have on more than a few occasions got my own words mixed up.

The police station at Methil had responsibility for the external security of the vastly expansive and partly underground warehouse complex owned by John Haig Distillery Group between the towns of Glenrothes and Markinch where occasionally officers were called when an intruder alarm was set off. There was a pre-determined procedure which required responding police vehicles to rendezvous at a number of fixed points. While this was being achieved, HM Customs and Excise staff accompanied by distillery personnel engaged on the premises conducted a full search within. As we awaited the result of the in-house security check on one such occasion an inspector at HQ came over the force radio network asking this sergeant if he could be of any assistance or was the matter under control? The sergeant proudly announced in his gruff Scottish brogue: 'Everything's under control sir, I've thrown an accordion around the premises.' The airwaves were vibrant for a few minutes with caustic comments, some sarcastic but mainly very funny and in keeping with a culture only truly understood by those who are part of it.

When Unit Beat Policing (now known as Community Policing, I believe) came to Fife, some of the instructions from HQ, of which there were many, were to be as visible as possible when patrolling the villages and towns. Personal radios were introduced to a limited number of officers, mainly drivers, the first issue of which was in two parts: a receiver and a transmitter. Both were about the size of a slim house brick and encased in rather naff blue plastic, hardly very robust, as time would tell. The transmitter had to be used with caution because when you depressed the transmit button the aerial shot out of the top of the device. You soon learned to keep it away from your eye or nasal area, for obvious reasons. When on vehicle patrol you were encouraged to park the marked 'Panda' car in a central and visible position, normally the market square or main street, and go walkabout. This was a combination of 'showing the flag' and meeting the Chief Constable's monetary constraints. I think we were restricted to 50 patrol miles per shift, excluding calls by the public to incidents. All well and good, but any local ne'er-do-wells would work out that once the Panda car was parked up and the officer set off on his foot patrol it would be thirty minutes or so before he would return, giving them ample time to get up to mischief. I understood the reasoning behind this, but it wasn't conducive to catching criminals so I adapted it somewhat, especially during night duty tours. When in areas where vehicle or burglary crime were prevalent I'd park the police car in a prominent place, but instead of walking about in normal uniform I would occasionally place my uniform cap in a duffle bag holdall favoured by miners, pull a 'donkey' jacket over my tunic and don a 'bunnet'. From afar I'd just look like a miner going to or coming from work.

This paid dividends one night when I heard the muffled sound of a car window breaking and from a point of concealment in a small town road I knew was a regular target for car thieves, I saw a couple of likely lads break into several cars and remove radios and other items from them, stashing their booty under another car parked nearby. While this was going on I radioed for assistance, requesting a silent approach, and guided the responding units into positions nearby. The two youths were stopped by the van crew as they were checking to see if the coast was clear or more likely looking for an expected pal to turn up with a car to take them and their goodies away. They were pretty cocky because they weren't in possession of their stolen goods. Both were known to us as burglars and car thieves. As we walked them back to the three vehicles I told them I'd watched them break into, they still denied any knowledge but when I showed them their stash hidden under another car, which happily (for me anyway) included a centre punch tool adapted for breaking car quarter lights, they realized that the game was up. This proved they had come out intent on theft and put their crimes up a notch or two above opportunistic theft. Neither wore gloves so fingerprints would probably convict them, coupled with my testimony. Their replies to my questions corroborated by my van crew colleagues were sufficient under Scottish law to arrest and charge them. They eventually admitted a number of other thefts from vehicles, so the CID was able to clear up a good number of unsolved crimes. The only slight downside to this good arrest was a sergeant I didn't know too well who arrived as we were recovering the stolen items and asked me why I was dressed as a miner. I tried to explain, but he simply told me not to do so again without permission. I was not CID, so I must be seen in uniform at all times. He didn't take it further so he was probably appreciative of my actions, but still felt he had to tell me to toe the party line.

Chapter 9

Time to Move On

I continued my day-to-day policing duties while awaiting a response from any of the law enforcement agencies I'd written to, having made up my mind to move on to another force, or even another country if necessary. It's fair to say that my preference at that time was, in fact, the RCMP. The first reply I received, however, was from the Met so I made the requisite arrangements to travel to London for an interview. First come, first served, after all.

I attended the Met's then recruitment office in Borough High Street in south-east London and went through a fairly lengthy selection procedure. After this I underwent a comprehensive medical examination then another more informal interview that covered such topics as the length of training course I would have to attend in order to be properly trained as an English PC. Because I was a serving Scottish PC I was informed that I would not need to go through the full initial training, but would need to learn the different powers of arrest, enactment of byelaws and other conditions of service that were required in an English police force which of course were slightly different to their counterparts in Scotland. I travelled back to Fife feeling quite confident that I would soon be serving in the Met.

Sadly this was not the case. Soon after my trip to London I was instructed to attend HQ to discuss my future prospects with one of the constabulary's senior officers. In effect I was submitted to a lecture incorporating the disappointment of the then Assistant Chief Constable (ACC) who remonstrated with me for abusing his constabulary budget plus Fife County Council taxpayers' money to obtain training and education as a cadet and then a PC, only to take this costly experience south to an English force. I was reminded of where my loyalties should be and asked to reconsider my decision. When asked why I wanted to leave, I somewhat nervously informed this rather imposing Victorian figure that I wished to specialize in the CID and wanted a more challenging career. I remember thinking I didn't want to wait forever for promotion which I knew and accepted in such a small force was pretty slow, but decided this probably wasn't the best forum or time to mention these concerns.

He proceeded to inform me that I could make detective constable 'within twelve years' if I kept up my current rate of progress. Twelve years is a bit more than a third of one's career, for goodness sake! This was one of the very reasons I needed to leave. Knowing he would not understand or accept my points of view, I kept my own counsel. He also inferred that the recent internal inquiry into the loss of cash from my locker might delay the transfer process because the Met would want to be assured that I was not to be charged with any criminal offence or be found guilty of any serious internal disciplinary offence before accepting my transfer request. He was correct in this regard.

After sticking to my request and confirming to the inspector at Methil police station that I would be continuing with my request to transfer to the Met, I was effectively sent to Coventry. In reality this meant being allocated all the miserable tasks and worst foot beat patrols in the meantime. I eventually sallied south after three years' service in Fife Constabulary. For the record, I loved my time with that force and it undeniably prepared me extremely well for the rest of my policing days. Ironically I am therefore of the opinion that Fife County Council's taxpayers' money and Fife Constabulary's budget was actually rather well spent.

As I was editing this section it was ironic that a day or so earlier I had read a newspaper article to the effect that certain English police forces were instigating a recruitment campaign encouraging applicants with no prior police experience to apply for direct entry into the CID. After a twelve-week training course they would become trainee investigators. My former Fife Constabulary ACC must have turned in his grave. After all, he had been offering me a CID post in twelve years, not twelve weeks. Apart from being plain daft, it's an insult to the many police officers still serving on the front line or in many of the other specialized roles, having earned their stripes so to speak by completing a two-year probationary period. My contacts still within the Met tell me that no-one wants to join the CID any more because of the abnormally high workload and continuous pressure from the courts and the CPS (Crown

Prosecution Service) surrounding disclosure of documents which, due to our society's reliance and abuse on social media takes up an inordinate amount of their time. You cannot simply train an investigator. The job has to be learned by experience on the street, on the beat, during investigations. You have to assess suspects and witnesses alike, analyse answers under caution from arrested persons and you need to learn police culture and procedure because there may come a time when you have to investigate bent police officers too. It's like asking for applicants to become jockeys when they've never ridden a horse. Or, to use another analogy, it's like any major football team only putting out a team of eight players instead of the normal eleven and then complaining because they lost the game. Absolutely ridiculous and naïve in the extreme. The public deserves better and was used to better.

No missive of mine would be complete if I failed to mention my good friend or, to use the Fife coal miner's colloquialism, my 'neeb', an abbreviation for neighbour and describing the miner you work with literally shoulder-to-shoulder on a daily basis and whom you trust implicitly. Former PC 122 John Muir, Fife Constabulary is my 'neeb'. I knew his dad who was a uniform sergeant in Dunfermline when I was a cadet there. Sergeant Muir was a very popular and respected individual, extremely smart in appearance which was probably a trait from his days in the Scots Guards and one that he handed down to John. As probationer constables John and I shared a number of experiences both professional and social, and shared a few scrapes and scraps while learning our craft. Initially we paired up through choice, but as our arrest returns grew the sergeants would deploy us together on a regular basis in order no doubt to get the best out of us. In a strange way I think some of our peers were pleased with this arrangement because they preferred a slower approach.

I'm proud to inform the reader that John is still the only police officer with whom I've shared an identity parade, as a suspect, that is! During the arrest of a drunken local waste of space who readily assaulted women and those weaker than himself and regularly caused breaches of the peace it was necessary to use appropriate and reasonable force when he kicked, fought and spat on us outside a local pub after having a bit of a disagreement with another drunk. He did receive a few injuries during the fracas, but neither John nor I had drawn or used our batons which we could have done and would have been justified in so doing because of his unnecessary aggression. There was a bit of a scuffle, ending up with us rolling around on the ground in order to place handcuffs on him to restrain him, which we eventually successfully accomplished. On arrival at the police station he complained to the sergeant that one of us had assaulted him inside the police van after he was cuffed and the doors closed. This was a total lie. He was examined by an on-call doctor who recorded his minimal facial bruising and treated a small cut to his mouth, then deemed him fit to be detained. Our hero appeared at court the following morning charged with disorderly conduct and assault on police and was bailed after tendering a not guilty plea.

Soon afterwards John and I were called into the inspector's office and informed that this individual had made a formal complaint of assault by us after being arrested and handcuffed and then, incredulously, the Insp asked us which one of us it was. We looked at one another as he repeated the question. John then told him the prisoner was lying and had not been assaulted in the police van, outlining that the injuries he received were caused during his violent resistance to being arrested. With an 'Okay, have it your way', he dismissed us.

Not long after that we were obliged to attend a formal ID parade in uniform after reiterating to the HQ officers tasked with investigating this allegation that it was fictitious to say the least. As is normal and legally accepted practice during ID parades involving police officers as suspects, our shoulder numbers were covered up. The complainant entered the room pushed by a friend in a wheelchair and was propelled in this manner up and down a couple of times before he stopped between John and me. He pointed to both of us, one after the other, and said: 'It was one of them. His number's 126.' The parade over, we were dismissed and told that we'd be informed of the outcome in due course. As he'd not picked the one responsible for this alleged assault but simply identified the only officers present during his arrest, we weren't unduly concerned. Allegations such as these made were/are commonplace against working cops so are not unusual. In the fullness of time he dropped this spurious allegation, shortly after he was found guilty as charged funnily enough. For the record John's shoulder number was 122 and mine 600. Somewhat spookily, when I later transferred to the Met the shoulder number I wore for the relatively few months I was in uniform was 126 (see photo plate section).

Chapter 10

Hendon it is then

The course at Hendon began well enough, especially when I discovered that my salary at the Met Training School was almost double that I'd earned in Fife Constabulary. Hendon was similar in many ways to Tulliallan Castle but with much less drill. Because of my experience as a former Scottish PC I was made class captain, which is akin to being a school prefect. In the absence of an instructor I had to ensure that the boys and girls were not late for tutorials and if necessary march them between classrooms and on occasions liaise between the class and training staff where required.

One of my first recollections from those Hendon days was that it was there I first heard the marvellous Bob Dylan song *Lay Lady Lay*. Not personally, unfortunately. A classmate who had attended the Isle of Wight concert earlier in 1969 played his copy of the concert on his cassette player each morning. Being a Dylan fan I really enjoyed this, but some of the other chaps were not too impressed. About a quarter of the intake were former Met cadets and a few, like myself, ex-cadets from other forces. A couple of guys were former soldiers. One who became a good pal nicknamed Wigan had been a semi-professional wrestler and another was the son of the Duchess of Sutherland who bore the title the Earl of Strathnaver. We knew him as just plain Alistair. Initially Alistair's presence brought a fair bit of media attention but he played it down and settled down to his studies and training programme just like the rest of us commoners.

I did have a bit of a problem with the uniform helmet, however. This is a singularly useless item of headgear in practical terms and less smart in my opinion than the cap bearing the readily-identifiable Sillitoe tartan that was pioneered by a former Glasgow City Police Chief Constable of that name who wished to distinguish his 'Polis' from bus conductors, postal workers and the like who were also adorned with dark blue caps. Incidentally, the British police and a large proportion of police forces in former Commonwealth countries later adopted the Sillitoe style. Yet another example of the very many Scottish innovations, by the way!

Chapter 11

Balham: A New Beginning

Upon successfully completing the Hendon course I was seconded to Wandsworth Common Police Station, 'W' Division, in the Balham area of south London (gateway to the south, according to the famous comedians The Goons), which was then mainly a working-class and predominantly Afro-Caribbean and Irish populace mixed with witty and gritty south Londoners. This offered me a great many more professional challenges than my previous police area in Fife. I also had to learn the local dialect, as indeed they had to try to fathom my Scots brogue. Each Met station is issued a phonetic code to aid with internal communications. The code for the 'nick' at Wandsworth Common was WC; phonetically 'Whisky Charlie'. My shoulder number was 126 WC. You can imagine the jokes spawned by this.

So here I was, like many Scots before me, seeking the London streets which were mythically claimed to be paved with gold. Fair enough. As far as I was concerned the Met would offer me more and greater challenges and opportunities to prove myself and hopefully specialize within my chosen career. The inevitable hard work would mean overtime payments; those would get me on the property ladder in due course which was a bonus. I'd driven down from Fife in a hired mini-van that contained virtually all the possessions of myself and my new bride, mainly wedding gifts. In pride of place was a lobster-pot stool with an orange-covered cushion, very trendy then. We'd been engaged for a while before I decided to leave our home county and were married after I completed the course at Hendon. The Met provided us with married quarters in the shape of a very acceptable two-bedroom apartment in Garrett Lane, Earlsfield in south London. Close by was a great little pub, a good Cypriot restaurant and a few streets away was the football stadium home of Wimbledon Football Club. What's not to like? My spouse soon obtained work in the Tooting branch of Marks & Spencer and I splashed out on a cheap and noisy French-made moped in order to travel the few miles to and from work. It was a start.

Not long after I began my new life, there I was on foot patrol in the Balham Hill area in uniform accompanied by a Special Constable. If any of you know the region you'll be aware, even if you don't want to admit it, that it was frequented in those days by 'ladies of the night' plying their services for sale in the oldest of professions, oft times referred to as a red-light district. It was regularly also used by them and their punters looking for business during the day.

Anyway, as we ambled along I heard and then saw a man and a woman arguing near the doorway of a large public house. They were both of West Indian appearance and I could not make out a word of what they were shouting about. We approached them to quieten things down, but immediately the bloke became quite agitated and directed his shouts at me while prodding me in the chest. Wearing the blue, as the term of being in police uniform is known, and firmly intent on upholding the fine traditions of the British Police in keeping the Queen's peace, I asked him to desist (in a Fife accent of course), which didn't make any difference at all, rather the opposite. I continued to enquire (naïvely in hindsight) after the lady's welfare, but the guy kept up his rant and pushed me in the chest again, this time more aggressively. Enough being enough, I then told him he was under arrest for assault upon me as well as a breach of the peace and then things really escalated. We struggled a bit but managed to restrain him and the Special was radioing for assistance when the 'lady' jumped on my back.

That was it. I drew my truncheon and handcuffs and, after sweeping the woman off my back, we cuffed the guy around a lamp post. I continued defending myself from this screaming banshee's antics by restraining her in a 'come along hold' which meant restraining an arm behind her back while holding her other shoulder pressed into the pub wall to avoid an elbow in the face when the cavalry turned up. One of them, Bernie Brown, is to this day still a good friend. The sergeant appeared bemused. Uppermost among his questions to me was the fact that as beat constables were not issued with handcuffs so obviously didn't carry them as part of their everyday kit in the Met in those days, where had I obtained the ones used to restrain the prisoner? I thought this a bit unusual considering the circumstances of the arrests and the fact that I'd been issued with and carried handcuffs from my first days in uniform in

Scotland. Still, rules are rules, or so they say. Of course I'd brought them from my old force as tools of my trade. At that time Met officers only carried handcuffs in certain fast-response vehicles. Otherwise they were stored in the desk sergeant's drawer at the local station from where they were issued, against signature of course, as and when required. A totally banal system, I thought. However, the sergeant thought differently and, after acknowledging my good work, advised me not to be seen carrying the cuffs in future, which advice I ignored in the belief that my safety and welfare were far more important than this ridiculous Met memo. Needless to say, my helmet had toppled off at the onset of this fracas and looked up at me uselessly from a south London gutter. My prisoner turned out to be a well-known pimp, wanted for non-payment of fines for previous brushes with the local magistrates, and of course his lady friend was 'on the game' as well as being suspected of thefts from some of her clients. Goodbye Lochgelly! Hello Balham!

After only eight months in uniform I was selected for plain-clothes duty as a Temporary Detective Constable (T/DC); basically an embryo detective. My progress in the Met was substantially far more accelerated than what I could have expected in Fife Constabulary for sure. I began working on the everyday street crime which affected every victim's life too regularly in that area, mainly trying to identify and then arrest pickpockets and other varieties of street criminals and started to build up a network of informants ('snouts'). Normally these were rather pathetic minor thieves, mostly with drug habits, whom no-one actually liked, including the coppers for whom they 'narked' (informed). Nevertheless, such informants are an essential tool for any detective.

I'd been chosen to join the CID in this capacity because I'd displayed more than a passing interest in local street thieves and burglars who were the scourge of the area and from whom the public deserved to be protected, and in seeing them get nicked. These arrests had obviously come to the notice of middle-ranking officers tasked with selecting suitable candidates for evaluation and training as future CID officers. T/DCs were still looked upon as uniform staff until eventually (and hopefully) selected as mainstream CID officers in due course. Not all made it, naturally. It was a rather precarious period in my career, but as I wanted to be a detective so much I was willing to give it my all to achieve this ambition. I soon noticed the difference working in plain clothes. Being able to walk or drive about without being identified as a police officer gave one more freedom to focus on the task in hand and not be distracted by other sometimes mundane demands of the general public that one attracted when in uniform. There was also the sense of elation and achievement when I 'showed out' (produced my warrant card) to an unsuspecting suspect of a stop and search procedure which proved successful or, even better, when effecting an arrest. I knew now that this was where I was meant to be as a copper.

I was paired up with a well-respected and experienced T/DC originally from southern Ireland named Billy Bourke. A soft-spoken, thorough but fair man, I learned a great deal at his side which would stand me in good stead later on in my professional career. He would sometimes interview suspected thieves and burglars for hours, talking about anything under the sun to gain their confidence and distract them from their lies or false alibis before extracting their confessions. Often we went through the station crime book (a record of burglaries/thefts reported in the area) page by page as if it were a sales catalogue with the suspect/prisoner who would in these instances occasionally indicate which crimes they'd carried out, which would very often lead us to the stolen goods and frequently more arrests. Billy shared cigarettes with them and provided copious amounts of tea during this procedure. How he regularly 'turned' hardened young thieves and apologetic victims of the system that failed to give them employment, respect, a future or decent housing I do not know, but I envied him this ability. Strangely enough, I think the villains simply trusted him, another trait that in my opinion is lost to us in today's police service. You can often learn a lot about a prisoner after their arrest which is not actually of any evidential use. Once charged, the prisoner is photographed, fingerprinted and antecedents noted for presentation to the court. During this process the individual can open up about their lifestyle and not unusually this is a time when they ask for favours such as bail or a good word from us to the magistrate to help them out. Why not? This was where Bill excelled. Quite a few 'tea leaves' (thieves) that we regularly nicked would refer to him as Mr Bourke which was undeniably due to their respect for him. Respect is a two-way street, so by giving them respect even while arresting them, they reciprocated. I made this a benchmark for myself.

In the station canteen fellow officers used to joke that he obtained confessions by simply boring the pants off prisoners with his continual questioning. I knew better. He was an astute and professional interrogator and a very shrewd judge of character. He often personally visited a mother or spouse of one of these characters and assured them that their loved one was okay while in police custody. By virtue of such humane gestures he was trusted by many criminals and their families alike and at the same time built up a large intelligence network in our 'manor'. It was not unusual while relaxing off duty in a local bar for a drink to be sent over to us from someone we'd arrested or questioned regarding some sort of criminality. There was a mutual respect then between certain types of criminal and the local Old Bill which regretfully I saw gradually diminish during my career.

To highlight this point I remember being told by a criminal I was processing that a few years earlier when he was serving yet another term in prison, a CID officer who was partly responsible for his incarceration was driving past this villain's apartment when he apparently noticed smoke coming out of a window. He stopped, alighted from his car and on approaching the front door he saw through a kitchen window that there was in fact a small fire so he kicked in the door and called out this villain's name in case any of his family was inside and maybe unaware of the fire. A neighbour appeared having heard the door go in and they both rushed in to check if anyone was about. It was apparently empty. The officer called the fire brigade who were on site very quickly and verified that no-one was at home. As the fire was extinguished, the villain's wife returned from shopping with their toddler. It became apparent that she'd left something on the cooker which had caught fire. This individual was amazed that the copper would take the trouble to check out his address, given that he was a 'tea leaf' and his missus a 'tom' (prostitute). In his mind he couldn't understand why any decent person would even try to help scum like him (his words, not mine). He was taken with the idea that his wife and child could have been at home and at risk of injury or even worse when my colleague had called in the fire. He was in his debt.

As a result he became a snout, although from time to time he inevitably returned to his thieving ways. Having said that, on the several occasions I dealt with him he was quite open and up front and accepted his lot. On one occasion I saw him drop a tenner into the Police Widows and Dependants' Fund collection tin that sat on the front desk after his personal property was returned to him as he left the police station on bail, having been charged with theft. I'm not sure if it was from the proceeds of crime or not, but in any case it was going to be used for a good purpose.

As previously mentioned, a T/DC's lot was to patrol the streets and with the use of selective stop-and-search powers arrest thieves and burglars or anyone else acting suspiciously. The luxury of an office desk was not for us. I recall a DS telling me shortly after I started that if he saw me in the nick I'd better have a prisoner in tow or an urgent need to use the loo, otherwise I'd be looking to return to uniform. We understood the rules and were fine with them. Keeping the streets as free from crime as possible was our goal. Regular and quality arrests were necessary to make substantive detective and we each knew there was a lot of competition among our peers to succeed. At the end of each month all T/DCs were summoned to the gym at Tooting Police Station where we would be addressed by the divisional DCS or his deputy and brought up to date on changing crime-fighting priorities, impending targets and changes in procedures. At the conclusion, the arrest returns of each of us were read out. We knew that if you were the bottom pair on this list and there was no particular reason for this, you had a month in which to improve your position or you would likely face a return to uniform duties. On one such occasion the two T/DCs who were named as bottom of the arrests list literally at the end of the meeting took to the streets with gusto to resolve their plight. Neither was ever in that position again and both went on to become substantive and, later on, promoted CID officers. I'm more than happy to report that neither Bill nor I ever had our names read out in this manner.

The most singularly and indeed significantly important book kept by every T/DC and in fact every CID officer at that time other than the pocketbook issued to every police officer was undeniably the CID diary. This, as the name implies, was a record of the hours of duty worked, a description of the work assigned, any expenses incurred (including payments made to informants) and, most importantly, at the rear a detailed list of arrests. This was the go-to or default document we all relied upon. It was a hard-backed blue book, the pages were enumerated and it was obligatory to complete each entry daily. It was submitted once a week for supervisory purposes and could be and occasionally was called to court, so its content was entered and taken most seriously. It was the yardstick by which supervisory DSs, DIs and ultimately the DCS assessed you. It was our life blood, so to speak.

For a period we were under the guidance and supervision of an experienced, and in the opinion of some colleagues, rather eccentric DS.

Apart from teaching and training us in elementary CID procedures and encouraging our thief-taking skills, he instilled in us an appreciation of fine wines and ports. Every now and again, by way of appreciation for our hard graft, we'd make a pleasant sortie across Battersea Bridge where he'd introduce us to friends of his who ran a couple of wine bars very popular in the King's Road area of Chelsea at that time; a part of my education that I thoroughly enjoyed and took to avidly.

More regarding this man's alleged eccentricity. While he was a uniform PC based at Croydon, during a night-duty foot patrol he popped around the back of a large department store where he unwittingly disturbed a couple of burglars attempting to enter the premises. A short struggle ensued, resulting in him being struck several times on the head with a crowbar being used by one of them to jemmy the doors open. The assailants got away. He was eventually found unconscious and not in a good state of health by colleagues searching for him after he'd failed to ring in as per normal from the police call box. This occurred prior to officers being issued with personal radios, so beat PCs had to ring in to their stations at regular intervals to keep in touch or make a report or alternatively were met by their patrolling sergeant at predetermined times and locations.

He was in hospital for some time in an induced coma and after a period was wheelchair-bound and undergoing recuperation and physio when 'the Job' decided that his head injury was so severe that he was probably not able to continue operating as a police officer due to cranial damage possibly affecting his decision-making and communication skills, not to mention his sanity. He was still a probationer at this time. He naturally disagreed and eventually obtained a certificate from a psychiatrist proving his sanity, dismissing the doubts the Job had mentioned in their dismissal proposal. He rightly won the medical appeal and was reinstated. From then on, when anyone questioned his sanity he'd produce this certificate, which he regularly carried on his person, as a disclaimer. He'd then usually invite the person to produce their own proof of sanity, which they rarely could, of course. To say the least he was a real character, but someone who taught me a great deal which stood me in very good stead throughout my career. In the interim the local CID had arrested and charged two men with this attempted burglary, grievous bodily harm to our colleague plus kindred other offences. Both were duly convicted and given substantial prison sentences for their misdeeds.

Section 4 of the Vagrancy Act 1824 was our bread and butter, commonly referred to as 'Sus' by criminals, police officers and lawyers alike. This was because if seen committing three consecutive suspicious acts such as trying vehicle door handles, walking up garden paths and looking into doors or windows of domestic or business properties, or following mainly females closely while looking into their shopping bags or handbags, the legislation allowed police to stop and question the individual and if necessary search them on the spot. Many an arrest was occasioned this way. Persistent offenders could be deemed 'incorrigible rogues' or 'vagabonds', making them liable to arrest simply if found in a public place. This legislation was brought in after the Napoleonic Wars when former soldiers often resorted to criminal endeavours in order to stay alive which, although tragic, could not be tolerated in a so-called civilized society. It still had a positive effect more than 100 years later. There's no doubt that these arrests prevented many a theft, burglary or mugging occurring, therefore helping to fight crime and make the London streets a little less threatening for potential victims.

I was gaining more responsibility with such enquiries and graduating through this important practical training. Eventually we snared a recidivist burglar who did not wish to go inside for a lengthy prison stretch so he volunteered to become an informant, which was not unusual in those circumstances. He was a fellow Scot so I was deputed as his 'handler' because even Bill had difficulty in understanding his rather guttural 'Jock' accent. He was charged with a token number of burglaries, which we could prove he committed, and granted bail in order to ferret around for information. This paid off when he soon informed on a gang of burglars and other criminals who dishonestly handled their produce, so we netted a fair few local villains and recovered a good deal of their victims' stolen goods, which is always a good feeling for any detective.

A couple of these victims of crime were a mixture of aspiring and established actors residing in the Chelsea and Battersea areas. I've often times seen them on TV or in films and recall those days when we shared the occasional beer or glass of plonk with them while obtaining a statement of evidence or returning their stolen belongings. It's a myth that officers in those days didn't partake of the occasional drink on duty by the way; well in the CID, that is, providing circumstances permitted.

One of these victims was the late Australian actor and comedian Bill Kerr. South African-born Bill was a stalwart in numerous Second World

War movies that were produced in the '50s and '60s in which he normally played a Kiwi or Aussie Air Force pilot or crew member, most famously in *The Dam Busters*. He also worked with some of the true maestros of comedy such as The Goons and Tony Hancock on their extremely popular radio shows. I met him when he reported a burglary at the bedsit he and his girlfriend occupied in the Nine Elms region of Battersea. He'd moved there from New York in order to help get a musical comedy onto the West End stage. It was set in the American Wild West at the end of the nineteenth century and was called *Liberty Ranch*.

One of the items stolen during this burglary was a large colourful 'ghetto blaster' stereo radio/cassette player which he'd brought from the US. He provided a couple of photographs of his apartment which showed this item in detail. There would have been very few of these items, if any, in London at that time. A couple of days later my colleague Bill and I were walking through a local housing estate on another enquiry when I spotted a youth with what looked like Bill Kerr's radio on his shoulder blasting out music. We tailed him unnoticed for a short distance as he knocked on a front door and then entered a flat. While I held the fort and kept lookout, Bill sought a search warrant and uniform assistance and upon his return we went in. To the surprise of said youth and a few of his mates inside we discovered other stolen items from Bill Kerr's burglary so a van was summoned, property was removed and a couple of ne'er-do-wells conveyed to Battersea police station 'to assist police with their enquiries'.

To cut a long story short, Bill Kerr positively identified the radio and other bits and pieces we'd recovered. After a couple of lengthy interviews Bill and I convinced the prisoners of the error of their ways and that the best thing for them and their future would be to admit their guilt. This they did, plus other similar burglaries in our area as we went through the major crime book. Other participants were implicated and searches of their addresses recovered even more stolen property. A very satisfying bit of work. Bill Kerr didn't manage to get *Liberty Ranch* into any West End theatre but I went to see a performance in Greenwich Theatre and thoroughly enjoyed it. Shortly afterwards Bill returned to the US and the next time I saw him was on celluloid playing an Aussie army sergeant in the epic war film *Gallipoli* starring a young Mel Gibson. Bill passed away in 2014 back in his beloved Australia.

Around this time some would-be anarchist tossed a home-made Molotov cocktail at the front door of the private residence of the then Metropolitan Police Commissioner Sir John Waldron, which caused only slight damage to the door but caused quite a flurry on the floors of Special Branch (SB) at New Scotland Yard. As a result the commissioner's personal security was increased, as was that of the Lord Chancellor Quintin Hogg, who resided a few streets away in a suburb of Putney. This security upgrade meant that armed SB or other armed police officers escorted these two dignitaries during their busy daily schedules and remained outside their respective homes until 2200 hours each day. From then until 0900 hours two 'W' Division T/DCs armed with no more than a short wooden detective-issue police truncheon and personal force radios patrolled in an unmarked CID car between these addresses with instructions to report any suspicious circumstances to the SB duty officer.

Bill and I were assigned to this duty on several occasions, during which we would occasionally park our unmarked Job Hillman Hunter car in front of the commissioner's residence, or that of the Lord Chancellor, and grab a bite to eat and a hot beverage from our thermos flasks. On more than one occasion Sir John would confront us and inform us that he didn't want or require such protection and that as we had much more important work to be going on with he'd ask us to leave. He was always most polite. He disagreed with the SB directive. We would equally politely concur with his instructions, only to leave and inform the SB duty officer by radio. Our report noted, the duty officer simply instructed us to return and continue security cover of both addresses as discreetly as possible. This happened on several occasions which, to say the least, we both found a bit boring, annoying and unprofessional. Obviously SB via the Home Office pulled rank on the commissioner in order to ensure the safety and security of both parties.

By way of contrast, early one Sunday morning we'd been parked up outside the Lord Chancellor's residence while also making the odd sortie on foot to check the commissioner's property when we saw Quintin Hogg walking towards us carrying an armful of newspapers and a large mug of tea or coffee. He wished us good morning as we alighted from our vehicle to greet him, then told us that his good lady was preparing us a hot breakfast. He bade us go inside his home and told us he'd sit in the CID car and catch up on reading the Sunday newspapers. We looked at one another, but before we made a decision he insisted we go and eat our breakfast before it got cold or we'd receive the wrath of his wife which, he added with a smile, could be formidable. I took a personal radio after showing the Lord Chancellor how to use the other one just in case anything happened and we went indoors and enjoyed a really good brekkie. After we thanked the Lord Chancellor and his wife for their kindness and returned to our protection duties Bill and I decided that this didn't require an entry in our duty log lest it should cause undue concern to the sedentary hierarchy in the secretive lair of SB at the Yard.

The elderly mother of a High Court Judge occupied an apartment in an expensive part of Battersea named Prince of Wales Drive and very close to Battersea Park. She'd responded to a knock on the door where she was confronted by a scruffy male who gave her some cock and bull story about looking for a friend's flat. Taking advantage of her being wheelchair-bound, he forced entry and then subjected the lady to a vicious assault while trying to find if she had any cash or jewellery on the premises. With the meagre contents of her purse and a few items he thought would gain him some cash he left her badly bruised and distressed. The CID attended and a description was circulated in which it was mentioned that the perpetrator looked like a tramp and smelled strongly of alcohol.

Knowing that certain areas within Battersea Park attracted this type of individual, Bill and I mingled around them and surrounding streets, pubs and cafés, in fact anywhere that someone of this ilk would congregate. We spoke with pawnshop owners and known fences (handlers of stolen property in the past) in Chelsea and Battersea who would sometimes inform on their clientele if it kept the Old Bill from looking too closely at their other daily business. Nothing positive was learned. We stopped and searched a couple of likely suspects, again to no avail. We let these individuals know that there would probably be a couple of bob available by way of reward and encouraged them to chat among their mates and see if they could provide any info that may help in leading to an arrest.

After a couple of days we suggested that it would be a good idea if we could interview the victim ourselves to see if she had recalled anything further now that she was recovering in safety and hopefully less distressed. The investigating officer (IO) agreed to this proposal. It's normal practice in any criminal investigation to go over an occurrence with a victim of crime after an initial interview. Occasionally their memory is tweaked and previously unmentioned details come to mind. After making an appointment through the family liaison officer (FLO) involved with this lady in order that she would know we were pukka, we went to see her. Over a cuppa she went through her ordeal and when we specifically dwelt on the physical description of her attacker she reiterated his clothing, approximate height, age, build, hair colour, perceived ethnicity, speech, and then to our utter surprise she mentioned an unusual tattoo on the lobe of his right ear. This tattoo had not been mentioned in her original statement.

We conducted searches at the Criminal Records Office (CRO) and local police stations and eventually turned up a name of an itinerant alcoholic with a history of minor crime. Currently he was of no fixed abode but a recent entry in Battersea police station intelligence records showed he'd been stopped in the vicinity a few days before as a result of a complaint about his drunken behaviour by a dog-walker in the park. He'd not been arrested as no offence was disclosed. Accordingly we redoubled our efforts in the same areas as well as chatting with some of the same potential informants we'd stopped earlier, but this time naming the suspect. After a day or so we again trawled the areas frequented by itinerants in Battersea Park and our determination paid off. We spotted the suspect. We talked with him, but he was too drunk to make any sense. We radioed for a uniform van and took him to Battersea nick where we alerted the IO who quite rightly took over the investigation of this suspect. Subsequently this waste of space admitted the assault and burglary, giving his alcoholism as mitigation. After pleading guilty he received a lengthy prison sentence which, apart from anything else, would hopefully help him break the hold that alcohol had over his behaviour. Bill and I received a commendation from the divisional DCS which was gratifying and would do our respective careers no harm at all.

I was confirmed as a substantive DC soon afterwards and transferred to another part of 'W' Division. By now my Fife brogue was Anglicized so I was better understood at all levels. I was dealing with more serious crimes, burglaries, serious assaults, sexual assaults and white-collar crime, as well as drug possession and dealing which sadly was becoming more and more prevalent and was impacting and in effect increasing street crime in the area generally. I mentored less experienced officers with potential to become detectives as I'd been mentored myself.

A not-so-memorable incident occurred one Sunday morning when I was catching up with the inevitable paperwork caused by police work and as a natural follow-on from arrests. I was busily writing up case files and compiling written statements of evidence for use in court as a result of a recent bout of arrests in which I'd been involved. I was in the CID office at Nine Elms police station for my troubles, it being quieter than the equivalent in the larger Battersea nick nearby. This small, old nick was situated near the much-loved Battersea Dogs Home. Around lunchtime a colleague and I walked the few yards to a pub on the corner near the railway bridge to grab a bite. As we reached the pub's front door I noticed a lot of activity in the railway sidings. A gang of about half a dozen blokes dressed in high-visibility tabards, some wearing hard hats, were operating a crane mounted on a low-loader parked in the street onto which they were loading railway lines and other kindred track equipment. Most appeared to be of Asian or Indian origin. Without further ado we went into the pub and had lunch. Leaving within the hour, all was quiet and the workmen and their equipment had gone. I returned to my paper-shifting and sedentary admin duties undaunted.

A few days later, still toiling through my backlog of paperwork within Nine Elms nick, a uniform PC brought a couple of guys upstairs into the CID office and introduced them to the duty DS. They were British Transport Police (BTP) CID officers. It became obvious during their chat with the DS that they were investigating a large-scale theft of railway lines. A ship docked in the Thames had been searched by HM Customs & Excise officers acting upon information received and a large amount of railway lines, BR heavy lifting equipment and other railway paraphernalia were discovered as the vessel prepared to sail to India. A number of arrests had been made. Apparently part of the stolen consignment had been removed from stock held in the BR Nine Elms region. Rather sheepishly and with slight embarrassment I interrupted their discourse and enlightened them as to my observations on that Sunday lunchtime. After making teas and coffees for all, I found myself having to compile yet another statement of evidence for the BTP officers.

Informant-handling took up a prominent part of my duties as I strove to cultivate them and draw upon their input. Eventually I was handling a quite prolific snout who was close to known and active armed robbers. As the level of information he provided grew, I knew that as a divisional CID officer I didn't have the expertise nor did division have the resources to deal with the alleged venture they were planning which allegedly involved the carrying and possible use of illegal firearms during an armed robbery. So after seeking counsel and advice from a helpful senior officer I passed the info to the experts at Scotland Yard. These experts were 'The Sweeney' as they were known in London criminal parlance: Sweeney Todd = Flying Squad (as in Cockney rhyming slang). They were portrayed extremely well in the very popular 1970s' cops and robbers television programme featuring actors Dennis Waterman and the late John Thaw. Quite literally the Flying Squad was a handpicked team of experienced, dedicated, courageous and highly-motivated detectives who dealt with organized and dangerous armed criminal gangs who had become the scourge of London at that time.

Referred to throughout the Met as 'the Squad', the Flying Squad was set up in 1919/20 when many disillusioned and disgruntled former soldiers came back from the Great War to find little had changed as far as their prospects were concerned, circumstances not dissimilar to their earlier contemporaries returning from the Napoleonic campaigns. They were faced with the reality of no jobs, little money and no apparent future. Firearms were easy to get hold of because a great number had been brought back from the trenches by squaddies as trophies. As organized and armed crime escalated, Scotland Yard formed this elite unit to combat this trend and investigate and arrest those involved. They were issued with former Royal Flying Corps (RFC) Crossley Tenders fitted with extensive aerials in order to communicate better and over greater distances. As the Squad's reputation grew and arrests added up, a national newspaper reporter was the first to refer to the unit as the Flying Squad because of these ex-RFC vehicles, and this nickname stuck. Incidentally the Flying Squad emblem is in fact a facsimile of the eagle emblem contained in the cap badge of the RFC, now the RAF.

The information obtained from this informant led the Squad to arrest a gang of men in two stolen vehicles, later found to contain face masks, a number of loaded handguns and shotguns as they waited in ambush for a cash-in-transit bullion van. Armed Squad officers ambushed them without a shot being fired or anyone injured. Several other known and hardened recidivists were swept up soon after these initial arrests, evidence having been found implicating them in support roles to their criminal buddies arrested in the street. The whole operation was a great success. The informant excelled himself and was rewarded accordingly. As his 'handler', I received the equivalent of being 'mentioned in despatches' for my professionalism in dealing with that part of the investigation, a first in my career and understandably one of which I was rightly proud.

Chapter 12

The Sweeney Days

Shortly thereafter, and much to my surprise, I was informed by my DI that a request for me to join the ranks of the Flying Squad had been approved by my DCS. I could not believe my good fortune. Me, a member of the elite Sweeney. All those long arduous hours on duty, social sacrifices of working weekends, public holidays and unsocial hours plus good old-fashioned endeavour had been worth it. As a T/DC you worked on average a six-day, sixty-three-hour week consisting of an eight-hour day followed by a thirteen-hour day repeated and normally fixed a month in advance. Sundays were normally taken as leave but if the need arose those could be cancelled as well. I recall getting the date of a thirteen-hour day wrong once after I'd booked tickets for my wife and me to attend a Rod Stewart concert. When I realized my mistake, I approached my DI, a dour Yorkshireman, and asked if I could just work eight hours that day. His response was simply: 'Do you want to be in the CID, lad?' Thankfully another T/DC pal swapped duties with me and we were able to enjoy the rather expensive concert. A posting to the Squad was undeniably the greatest aspiration and achievement of most Met detectives then, therefore competition was fierce and only accomplished by a few. So just over three years after transferring from Fife Constabulary where my ACC had rebuked me for in his opinion abusing Fife taxpayers' funding to learn my trade only to walk away from the chance of becoming a DC in twelve years there, I was not only a substantive DC in the Met now but soon to be a member of the renowned Flying Squad. Beat that, ACC...with respect...Sir!

At that time twelve separate squads made up the Flying Squad each led by a DI, other team members being DSs and DCs with highly-trained PC drivers in support. I became part of 8 Squad based at New Scotland Yard. Within Squad parlance we were known as the 'Dip Squad' because half the team specialized in arresting professional and persistent pickpockets, especially international organized teams that targeted London, and the term 'dip' being London slang for a pickpocket. We regularly arrested home-grown dip teams too. Having no longer to be suited and booted (wear a suit, collar and tie) every day, usually only for court purposes now, felt good and was more comfortable. The more casual, in fact scruffier, the better from now on then. After intensive surveillance training I joined the rest of the team working the London Underground system, streets surrounding Harrods department store, Regent Street and Oxford Street areas where wealthy targets abound, Wembley football stadium, Buckingham Palace and many other locations where crowds gather for a particular event and we knew would attract such criminals especially during the summer months. I recall taking a much-needed mid-morning break from combing the streets around Harrods for dips by partaking of a coffee and croissant in the Food Hall in Harrods. Here was I not that long after transferring from Fife polis where I would take the odd tea break in a coalminers' canteen or High Street bakery enjoying a tea break in probably London's poshest and world-renowned departmental store in Knightsbridge. I had to pinch myself.

One morning I was travelling in a covert vehicle with a couple of colleagues on our way to set up an observation post on an active team of dips we had identified operating in some of these venues. As we drove down Buckingham Palace Road our attention was drawn to a bit of a scuffle on the rear platform of a red London bus directly in front of us. Suddenly a youth leaped off and began running down the pavement at speed. The bus came to a swift halt and we saw a couple of young back-packing females of Mediterranean appearance run after him. Our driver pulled up ahead of the fleeing youth and two of us jumped out to confront him. When he spotted us he slowed down and quickly tossed a wallet or similar item over the high wall to his left. We grabbed him and as we showed him our ID the chasing females caught up. They were in an agitated state but quickly calmed down when they realized that we were plain-clothes police officers.

It transpired that the youth had nicked a wallet from one of the girls' back-packs. Of course, this was what he'd thrown over the wall when we blocked his escape. The girls were in fact serving Israeli soldiers on leave touring the UK. He was probably a lucky boy in that they hadn't caught up with him. When challenged with this allegation, he simply shrugged his shoulders. In order not to show out our mode of transport we summoned a uniform van and all were taken to the local nick. Sure enough, enquiries revealed that our boy was a persistent dip. The girls were due to return to Israel the following day and the stolen wallet contained, among other items, the military ID and passport of one of them. We now had a bit of a problem concerning the recovery of this wallet. The wall that we'd seen it thrown over was in fact a wall surrounding the rear of Buckingham Palace:

- Was HM The Queen in residence?
- If so, could I ask her if I could have a rake around in her back garden please ma'am?

Seriously though, it was a concern. I contacted the Duty Officer in charge of the Met uniform unit responsible for security within the Palace and briefed him on the arrest. I informed him of the requirement to recover the wallet as soon as possible, not only for evidential purposes but to facilitate the flight home of the Israeli soldier. I described in detail the exact spot where it had been thrown over. Understandably he declined my offer to help his officers to search the area but confirmed that he'd have someone take a look there as soon as duties allowed. Within a short period of time this fine chap got back in touch, his staff having found it.

The Israeli soldiers made their way home as required and our dip 'ducked his nut' (pleaded guilty) the following morning before a stipendiary magistrate and received a suitable custodial sentence. We joked afterwards about what would have happened if the Royalty Protection Inspector had refused our request and I'd appeared before the stipendiary magistrate at the local court requesting a search warrant to recover 'known stolen property from the garden of an address of a Mrs E. Windsor in Buckingham Palace Road, SW1'. Your guess is as good as mine.

Organized international pickpocket gangs were the scourge of central London at this time, but even more of a problem was the ever-increasing blight of armed robbery upon cash-in-transit bullion vans. Another Flying Squad team had successfully identified a team of London bank robbers who specialized in this field of criminal endeavour and had arrested a number of them, recovering an abundance of evidence. These colleagues had also succeeded in 'turning' one of the main participants into what is described in police parlance as a resident informant, better known to the public as a super-grass (a nickname created for such criminal informants by a reporter on a national newspaper), and as a result of his admissions and written testimony literally dozens of other dangerous and serious recidivistic criminals were being arrested. The press had a field day with the revelations of this informant whose name was Maurice O'Mahoney, known to his mates as Mo. It didn't take long for a reporter to come up with the tag 'Mo the Grass'.

DS Alec Edwards, a proud Welshman, and I from 8 Squad were assigned to this team which operated out of Chiswick police station in West London where Mo was held pending de-briefing, albeit technically in prison custody. We initially assisted with regular armed escorts of dozens of these individuals to and from the local magistrates' court, police stations and prisons. Several others named by Mo were similarly granted resident informant status and held in other nicks nearby. Alec and I were tasked to look after one of these less dangerous criminals who had allegedly been an unarmed getaway driver on a couple of armed robberies but didn't take part in any form of violence. He was of previous good behaviour too, which was unusual. He insisted that when he saw one or two of his mates making a lot of easy money carrying out these blags he eventually succumbed because he was in a bit of debt and struggling to find enough money for he and his wife and family to enjoy life while working long, hard hours in the building industry.

During his de-briefing we'd occasionally take him out of his cell for a bit of a run around Richmond Park or other similar venue in order to give him some exercise and fresh air. He would have been entitled to regular physical activity had he been held in prison, but there was no such facility in the nick where he was held in safe keeping. I was quite fit in those days so I'd don a track suit and trainers and run alongside him while Alec and our driver, the legendary late Jim Moon, crept along behind us in a squad gunship. I also comfortably concealed my Smith & Wesson snub-nose detectives' special revolver in my underarm shoulder holster, just in case. Our charge and I got on quite well under the circumstances as we jogged along and chatted about a variety of subjects. On several occasions after we'd completed our run we'd take him to a 'greasy spoon' café where he could indulge in a full English breakfast as a bit of a treat. Food at the nick was nothing to write home about. He was well aware that if he tried anything stupid while being accorded these privileges he would not only lose the facility but might find his resident informant status revoked, meaning he'd be returned to prison where he would be in extreme danger from criminal associates of those against whom he was about to give court testimony.

I had always found court work fascinating. I found the thrust and parry 'twixt briefs (lawyers) and police officers stimulating and fascinating. It was almost theatre at times as a few nasty briefs tried any trick in the book to get their client off. It was almost a confirmation of guilty involvement of a prisoner when they asked for a certain named brief to be contacted. We were well aware of a small group of briefs who were in receipt of financial retainers from recidivistic professional criminals to represent them whenever they were arrested. The late Michael Worsley QC was one of Britain's most experienced and distinguished criminal lawyers who represented the Flying Squad in many armed robbery cases and he once referred to these lawyers and attorneys 'as of the alternative Bar' in a trial in which I was involved at the Central Criminal Court, or Old Bailey as it is generally better known to the public.

In a five-handed armed robbery trial at Snaresbrook Crown Court I was giving evidence of arrest and resultant interviews which had already stretched over a couple of days. Each defendant had his own brief. One of them was singularly unpleasant and made a number of insidious allegations against me and my fellow officers which ranged from 'being a stranger to the truth' as well as 'concocting and falsifying his client's answers to police during interviews' and the almost ubiquitous 'planting of weapons'. During a lengthy verbal attack outlining my allegedly corrupt and untrue testimony a wasp began buzzing around me in the witness box which was a bit of a distraction. The judge who sat close to the witness box noticed it and bade an usher fetch an aerosol spray to remove it. Apparently it was not unusual at that time of year in these courtrooms which were of a temporary nature as renovations were being carried out in the main building. After a few minutes as the brief continued his rant at me the wasp returned and flew around and very close to my head. I was trying to avoid it while forming a suitable response in my mind to one of his nastier questions when he reached across the front benches, removed his wig and threw it over to me, saying words to the effect that 'this might help'. To his regret I was paying attention to the wasp and not to his antics so the wig flew straight into my face. There was a hush in the court. Some of the jurors looked appalled, others bemused. The judge immediately called a halt to proceedings and instructed the jurors to take a ten-minute break. I could see the other defence counsel shaking their heads, realizing that this incident had not helped their cause. Some shared a few words with their humbled colleague, which didn't seem to be supportive as his wig was returned to him by the court usher and he meekly replaced it on his head.

The judge remonstrated with the offending counsel, describing his behaviour as inexplicable and disrespectful. He instructed him to apologize to me upon the return of the jury and then apologize to the court for his actions. Counsel maintained that the wig had slipped out of his hand. He had not meant to throw it, but he thought I was using the wasp's presence to buy time to create an answer or otherwise deliberately avoid answering his questions. As a result he'd become annoyed. The judge reminded counsel that any witness avoiding replies to questions was his responsibility and not that of counsel. He then kindly asked me if I was okay and was I satisfied with his handling of the incident. I acquiesced in the content. Court-speak for 'I'm fine thanks'.

When the jury returned, suitable apologies were made by this counsel as directed. To my amazement he then grumpily and sheepishly sat down, saying: 'I've no further questions for this witness.' I wouldn't be human, and in fact would have been a stranger to the truth, if I hadn't had a little chuckle to myself at the obvious embarrassment of this arrogant, supercilious prat. At the conclusion of the case the jury found all five defendants guilty of conspiracy to commit robbery and possession of firearms. All received substantial custodial sentences because all had previous serious criminal convictions (pre cons). One of the defence counsel who I knew from other trials told me during a subsequent court case that his colleague's antics had undoubtedly tarnished their case in the eyes of the jury. He said he and fellow counsel felt the mood of the jury swung towards the prosecution after the outburst, which was apparent due to the nature of the questions they asked of the judge prior to being sent off to deliberate.

It was at times enlightening when reading out the pre cons in court proceedings to see the look on some jurors' faces. You could read relief in some and could make out surprise in others when they heard the defendant's past transgressions. I also enjoyed the buzz when identifying myself as a Flying Squad officer. The jury normally appeared to take more notice, especially when firearms were part of the evidence. Unfortunately, because of the failings and criminal actions of a few former Flying Squad members you had to get used to regular allegations of corruption as well. It came with the job, I'm afraid. However, one aspect I could never come to terms with after receiving a roasting in the witness stand and the jury finding for the prosecution was defence counsel offering me his hand afterwards and saying words to this effect: 'Nothing personal, officer. It's all in a day's work.' It's one thing to test the evidence to the nth degree but another to try to discredit the witness needlessly, in my considered opinion.

At around this time *The Sweeney* television series featuring the late John Thaw and Dennis Waterman was in its infancy. For a couple of weeks before the pilot episode was screened these actors were given liberal and unprecedented access to the Squad offices at the Yard, driven around in some of our powerful unmarked Squad cars as well as being briefed on Squad parlance and everyday workings; in essence shown a day in the life of the real Sweeney. As their presence became more regular and they both acted quite normally, we pretty much became comfortable with them around, so much so that on one occasion a DI was a few minutes into a briefing for an early-morning armed raid to be carried out the following day, hopefully to apprehend a wanted felon, when it was pointed out to him that Dennis was sitting at the back of the room reading through some notes. The actor was diplomatically asked to join his crew in another room, which he did with a wry smile on his face. He was a natural in the role, as was John Thaw.

The circulation of this popular programme included broadcasts to British military personnel stationed in Germany via the British Forces Broadcasting Service (BFBS). As a result it was also seen by German civilian viewers who became very interested in the real Sweeney. A director from one of that country's national TV companies was given permission by the then Commissioner Sir Robert Mark to film a fly-on-the-wall documentary of the Squad at work. It was agreed that an actual ambush and arrest of three armed robbers as they attacked a cash-in-transit vehicle in a south London street several years earlier would be the crux of the programme. In Squad-speak this is known as 'a pavement job', normally a very rewarding and exhilarating, albeit dangerous conclusion to a lengthy and demanding information-gathering and surveillance operation.

Because of our casual, or some might say rather unkempt or even scruffy appearance, two other 8 Squad members and myself were chosen

74

to portray the bad guys and 1 Squad personnel were to be the arresting team. Over the next couple of days we three – ironically an Englishman, a Scotsman and an Irishman – were filmed in Soho bars and strip clubs under the surveillance of 1 Squad officers as we planned our 'criminal venture'. We were 'tailed' (followed) obtaining a stolen car displaying false plates and collecting a 'happy bag' (colloquially a bag of illegal firearms, masks and body armour to be used in a robbery).

On the big day, in fact evening because the real attack took place just after midnight in the street outside a south London Post Office sorting office, one of the generators used by the film crew to light the scene broke down. During the wait for a replacement, some bright spark in the film crew decided that a few bottles of beer would help to pass the time. When shooting commenced (i.e. the film, not discharging firearms), the alcohol may have had an adverse effect on some of the arresting officers because we three bad guys received more than a few bruises during our fruitless attempts to resist arrest. Thankfully the arresting officers' firearms were loaded with blanks, as were ours. This was my one and only brush with acting, I'm pleased to say. The German director was delighted with the outcome and apparently it was well received by his national audience too.

Chapter 13

Promotion: Onwards and Upwards

The 1970s were a particularly busy time in my life and career. In 1976 I was promoted to DS which was a bit of a double-edged sword situation as I was more than pleased to become a detective sergeant, but it meant that I had to leave the Flying Squad because there was no vacancy for a DS in their ranks at that time. Such is life. I was transferred to 'C' Division, which covered a large expanse of central London and brought me another raft of challenges and opportunities. I was initially based at West End Central, then the historic Bow Street police station where, apart from general CID duties, I took responsibility for running the Crime Squad and helped to train selected uniform officers endeavouring to become fully-fledged detectives, just as I had done.

In September 1977 I became a dad for the first time with the birth of a lovely wee daughter who we named Lorna. It was time to celebrate a new life and put to one side the sadness, dissatisfaction, grief and distress that pretty much had filled my working days for a while and look towards a bright future.

Several weeks later at the start of a day shift I was trawling through the major crime book noting details of overnight burglaries that I'd be obliged to attend with a SOCO (Scenes of Crime Officer) to investigate further after night-duty officers had recorded the initial findings. I noted that one victim was a Mrs K. Crosby. Thinking nothing more of this, I continued to prepare my list of visits when the DI walked in and, after ascertaining that I was covering these burglaries, told me that the 'Guvnor' wanted to see me pronto, the Guvnor being the Detective Chief Superintendent (DCS) in charge of all 'C' Division CID officers.

I duly popped up to his office where I saw that he had a copy of a burglary crime sheet on his desk in front of him. He politely bade me sit down and after a few pleasantries asked me what arrangements I'd made regarding Bing's burglary. It was then that the penny dropped.

I hadn't made the connection. After a brief chat he told me he would be going to the recording studio in west London where Bing Crosby was re-recording his famous and still popular *White Christmas* album to interview the great man. I was to leave no stone unturned at the address of the burglary where I would meet Bing's wife Kathy. The DCS was a great Guvnor and a highly-respected detective, but I'm not aware of any other DCS during my service who became involved in a basic burglary enquiry. Call me old-fashioned, but I could have dealt with it quite adequately. At the end of the day, however, he was the Guvnor.

I met and interviewed Kathy Crosby and their butler while the duty SOCO carried out a detailed forensic examination at the house they'd rented. Among items stolen was a pair of unique gold candlesticks that Kathy had commissioned as a surprise present for Bing. I subsequently visited the Hatton Garden jeweller who had manufactured them and obtained a photograph of same which I circulated locally and internationally via Scotland Yard's Arts & Antiques Squad. Sadly, very shortly afterwards Bing Crosby suddenly and unexpectedly passed away.

A month or so later I was contacted by an officer of the International Criminal Police Organization (ICPO) in Paris, better known to the public as Interpol, to the effect that New York City police officers had recovered the candlesticks from a jeweller in Manhattan. As I began making arrangements to travel to New York to obtain witness statements and recover the items, I was informed by the Yard travel section that a couple of Scotland Yard Arts & Antique Squad officers were already in New York on enquiries of another nature so they would cover my enquiry for me. Bugger. I'd never been to the US at that time. When my colleagues brought the items to me I took them back to the jeweller who'd made them and had them positively identified. As no person was ever identified as having stolen them, they were eventually returned to Kathy in the US.

Bow Street was a fascinating old nick. On the odd occasion when it was quiet in the wee small hours of night duty, especially during warm summer evenings, I used to walk around in tourist mode during my meal break, with my personal radio in my pocket just in case, often taking in the back streets of the marvellously historic City of London. Theatre-land, Soho and Covent Garden areas especially intrigued me. On one of these sorties I walked up Bow Street returning to the CID office when I noticed a group of three men sitting on the steps of the magnificent old

Royal Opera House building which sits directly across the road from where Bow Street nick stood. Sadly this fine old Victorian nick is part of a hotel complex now. What a pity that the establishment gave up on the fascinating and intriguing history of both the old nick, where Sir Robert Peel's new police force began, and the Magistrates Court next door, which could tell a tale or two about the famous and notorious rogues such as Oscar Wilde who passed through its chambers. Anyway, going back to my spotting these three chaps, I saw that they were chatting quietly and passing a bottle between them. As I drew closer, considering whether to have a word with them or not, I recognized them as none other than a trio of fine popular actors namely Peter O'Toole, Richard Harris and Oliver Reed. I accorded them a brief nod and went on my way, leaving them to their thespian chit-chat or whatever.

Digressing just a little, I'm proud to own a limited edition of a print produced to commemorate 150 years of London's detectives which photographically depicts the original officers of Peel's new police (aka 'Peelers') in their fine uniforms as well as in various disguises as hackney carriage drivers, down-and-out ex-soldiers, vagrants and tradesmen. Very impressive. The inscription is also most impressive:

> When in 1842 eight Metropolitan Police Officers were allocated to detective duties no-one could have foreseen that they would be the embryo of what was to grow into today's detective force. The worldwide reputation of Scotland Yard detectives has been hard won, richly deserved and carefully nurtured. For many years Scotland Yard detectives travelled the country, and still travel the world, to help solve complicated and/or sensitive crimes. At the root of all this remains the detective – highly motivated, highly skilled, heroic at times, dogged and determined in the highest tradition of the Metropolitan Police.

At least that used to be the case. This fine print bears the signatures of the first Joint CID Commissioner Richard Mayne (1842) and Commissioner Sir Peter Imbert, QPM (1992).

Incidentally, the not very well-known reason that the glass on the police lamps outside what used to be Bow Street Police Station were white and not the traditional blue was at the insistence of HM Queen

Victoria, who was a regular visitor to the Royal Opera House which, as mentioned earlier, was situated directly opposite. She demanded that they match the white of those outside the theatre. She was the queen, after all.

On another warm, quiet summer's evening I was cruising through the mews and back streets of central London in an unmarked CID car along with another night-duty detective on random patrol 'looking for murder and arson and drunks as they strolled down the street', to quote a line from a Billy Connolly song concerning Glasgow's finest. A taxi immediately in front of us in a narrow mews suddenly braked to a halt and a male occupant jumped out, took a few steps – jumps, even – and kicked open a house door, then ran upstairs. Thinking he'd 'bilked' (avoided paying) the fare, I showed out to the cabbie only to find out that the guy had not only paid his fare but given the happy cabbie a substantial tip.

There was a bit of a din coming from the first-floor front room of the house this guy had entered. Windows were open, loud music could be heard and shouting began between a male and female within. As I opened my car door to continue patrolling, a large object flew out of this open window and crashed on the cobbles below at the same time that a female screamed. We saw the item was a now broken record player. Deciding to intervene, we ran up the same stairs, found the door at the top ajar so ran in, warrant cards displayed. We were confronted by a very attractive young female hugging, as if trying to console, a guy who had his back to us. There was a bit of disarray in the room and most strikingly facing us near the door stood a very big bloke, and I do mean a very big bloke. Too much time spent chucking weights around in the gym and probably too much steroid ingestion, I pondered. He checked our ID, then politely asked: 'What's the problem officer?' I began telling him what we'd seen and heard when the guy being hugged turned around. I was looking straight into the face of the legendary Keith Moon. I couldn't believe my eyes. To say the least, I was/am a fan of the fabulous rock band The Who. It turned out that this was his pad so the record player would be his too, no doubt. The female was obviously a girlfriend and the very big bloke probably a minder. After a short chat including a sort of apology from The Who drummer who (no pun intended) had probably partaken of a little more of 'what made Milwaukee famous' than he ought, we departed after I diplomatically advised all that the matter would rest here, providing police were not called to any further disturbance. The minder cleared up the debris in the street as we drove off. 'Talking 'bout my generation...' You'll of course be aware, dear reader, that sadly in 1978 this brilliantly talented musician but flawed individual died of a drug overdose. Such a great loss...

It was time to take baby Lorna to Fife to show her off to family and friends who couldn't make the trip to London to see her. I took some time off during this visit to grab a couple of hours with some of my former Fife police pals at a favourite tippling hole of ours known as the Golf Tavern in Leven, a fine seaside town and popular holiday resort, especially with golfers, situated near to where I'd been stationed in Methil. While chatting, one of my buddies asked if I'd heard about the police dog-handler who'd been arrested for burglary and thefts a while ago. This was the same PC who'd informed HQ CID of my purchase of a Mini car which I'd obtained via a part-exchange deal and an additional payment of £80 during an internal investigation into my loss of £80 from a drowned victim that caused me a great deal of grief while I was still with Fife Constabulary. It transpired that the dog-handler had been caught in the act of committing a burglary and had subsequently admitted several others. He asked for a number of other thefts to be taken into consideration (TIC) in order, no doubt, to reduce his sentence. One of the TICs was the theft of the £80 cash from my locker. I was flabbergasted, not a little disappointed, and then downright angry. This dishonest cop had been interviewed at length, convicted and was quite rightly serving a prison sentence, yet no-one either in the court service, nor more importantly to me in Fife Constabulary, saw fit to inform me. As far as I was concerned I was still a suspect. I expected more. In point of fact I deserved more. I felt that at the very least a simple phone call, officer to brother officer, would have covered it. Well, at least the matter was finally resolved and I was vindicated of any dishonesty.

Chapter 14

The 'Maltese Mafia'

The following year I was engaged in extensive investigations to break the hold that the so-called 'Maltese Mafia' had on prostitution, pornography, illegal gambling and money-laundering in London's West End. A number of main players had been rounded up, interviewed at length, then charged and were awaiting trial on serious criminal charges. Others had flown the coop. The guvnor (a fellow Fifer who was my DCI) decided that I should go get them while the rest of the investigation team carried on with local enquiries because I'd done a fair bit of work on these individuals and knew many of them by sight as well as by reputation. I was linked up with another DS who had a Fraud Squad background and, suitably armed with a *commission rogatoire*, we flew to our first stop in Milan to obtain evidence to arrest and charge these absconders where necessary and ideally have them extradited to the UK if possible to stand trial with their peers.

A *commission rogatoire* is an internationally-recognized legal document, basically a Letter of Request signed by the UK's most senior legal officer to his/her counterpart in the country involved and which has to be lodged in that country's Supreme Court so that law enforcement bodies there are given the necessary authority to assist UK officers, as requested within the wording of the document, with either tracing witnesses or arresting perpetrators. A Maltese national citizen holding a bank account outside of Malta without disclosing same to the Maltese authorities committed a criminal offence then, hence the need for me to be accompanied by an officer with banking and criminal fraud experience to explain the detailed fiscal dealings of the suspects we sought to the Maltese authorities.

The Italian equivalent of the Flying Squad, exquisitely named the *Squadra Mobile*, assisted us in tracing and interviewing several suspects in Milan who it was our intention to use as witnesses against the main mafia members awaiting trial in London where possible.

About a week later we flew to Malta for the main part of the enquiry and were met there by DI George Grech who would be our liaison officer during our stay. George subsequently became a personal friend of mine and would also become the first Maltese national Commissioner of Malta Police. He subsequently became heavily involved with Scotland Yard's intriguing and tragic Lockerbie bomb investigation after it was established that the Samsonite suitcase containing the bomb responsible for bringing down Pan Am Flight 103 in 1988 was believed to have also contained baby clothes of Maltese origin (although God knows how they weren't destroyed in the explosion and subsequent crash). These were traced to a Maltese merchant who became one of the main prosecution witnesses in terms of endeavouring to identify the bomber.

Our time in Malta was fascinating and extremely interesting and I learned a great deal as an investigator as a result. Sinisterly, however, our rooms in the fine old Dragonara Hotel which was our place of residence and our hire car were 'turned over' (searched) one evening by persons who made no attempt to cover up their search, presumably friends of those we sought, as we took a much-needed break and meal with George and his family. No doubt they were looking for the bank details of their associates which they assumed I'd brought from London to aid our investigation. However, I'd sensibly secured these in the safe of the commissioner of the Malta Police at their HQ in Valletta on arrival. Apart from the obvious, this was particularly disconcerting because we'd booked into the hotel and hired the private motor vehicle using pseudonyms. We assumed a prepared legend – in layman's terms a false identity and job description – should we need to explain our presence in Malta to anyone other than those in the know. This is normal practice when working abroad where there's an element of personal danger necessitating covert surveillance or other forms of confidential police enquiries. In our case we would claim involvement in the withdrawal of HM Royal Navy staff and naval craft that were due to return to the UK and which was actually occurring at that time. Due to this unfortunate breach of security we were expeditiously moved to a far more secure five-star hotel for the remainder of our stay, and a very grand hotel it was too.

One evening George took me to a small bijou bar in the holy city of Mdina which was owned by a former police sergeant friend of his.

Mdina is a beautiful medieval place, formerly the capital of Malta and frequently referred to as the Silent City. We were there to watch a televised Manchester United football game as George was aware of my being a fan. As we talked, the owner's wife kept popping through beaded curtains behind the bar where I could see her preparing food on a small three-ringed gas cooker. After tasting a couple of these flavoursome dishes, which I thought were akin to Spanish tapas, her husband asked if I'd decided which meal I wanted. She was apparently giving me tasters of their limited menu and not doing tapas. Oops! I chose one, apologized for my naïvety, and bought us all a large glass of local red wine. As we replenished our glasses and settled down to watch the match, the street door opened and a Roman Catholic cardinal fully bedecked in a red cassock and cap, including a Manchester United scarf around his neck, entered. He'd been the local priest in Mdina when George was a uniform inspector there and used this bar as his local then so everyone present knew him. He was visiting the current priest and on learning that the Manchester United match was being televised he'd come to watch the game too. Not surprisingly, I think his presence limited the vocabulary and responses of the other fans in the bar as a goal was missed or a foul committed. After the match he invited George and I back to the priest's residence for a nightcap of fine Irish whiskey. His depth of knowledge of football and Manchester United in particular was commendable.

While we were working away in Malta the head of the Roman Catholic Church, His Holiness Pope John Paul I, died suddenly. This sad event meant that Malta, being a predominately Roman Catholic country, went into mourning. Two days of public holiday were declared so my Fraud Squad colleague and I had to revert to tourist status because our liaison officers took leave. Not too difficult for us in this wonderful holiday island. The majority of the individuals we sought were steadfastly identified and traced, both in Malta and the nearby smaller beautiful island of Gozo, then brought in for interview by George's team in our presence. As expected, many were known to the Maltese police as petty criminals.

To interview one of these individuals we travelled by means of an old flatbed ferry the short sea distance of approximately twenty minutes duration from Malta to Gozo. En route about mid-distance between these islands a shoal of flying fish suddenly emerged from the starboard side and flew over the low deck railings where quite a number of them landed on the deck, clattering and writhing around. Nearly all the somewhat elderly lady foot passengers dressed in traditional black dress and headscarves favoured by Maltese widows swiftly got among the thrashing fish and scooped up as many as they could into their pinafores. It was an incredible sight. These migratory Dorado fish are to be found in these waters in autumn and are known locally as *lampuki*. A crusty pie made with these fish is a Maltese delicacy which I tasted several times during my stay and thoroughly enjoyed.

We were met at the Gozo ferry terminal by a uniform police inspector with whom we walked the short distance to his office which had been the residence of the former O/I/C of the Royal Marine contingent when Britain held a military presence here. It was truly bizarre, to say the least, that on this pleasantly warm day as we sat in the inspector's office sharing a cold beer while discussing strategy, with the knowledge that an individual who had been arrested at our behest awaited interview in the cells below our feet, I was watching a group of nuns from the convent situated next door, dressed in full regalia, plucking oranges from fruit trees in a small orchard grove to the rear of the premises. The Maltese police work in their own indefatigable way.

One evening George very kindly invited us to a formal dinner in the Maltese government building so we hired appropriate attire and attended. We were introduced to a number of Members of Parliament and other dignitaries over pre-dinner drinks and just before taking our seats at the dining table we were led out to a balcony of this splendid old building which overlooked the great harbour of Valletta to witness the final withdrawal of the Royal Navy from Malta. The Maltese Socialist Prime Minister Dom Mintoff was no friend of the UK and had begun to expel British troops in 1978. As we watched the aircraft carrier HMS *Ark Royal* with her immaculately-uniformed crew lined up in whites along the decks to a Royal Marine band playing military marches slowly sail out escorted by a few other Royal Navy warships of the line, I noticed a couple of the more mature Maltese politicians with tears in their eyes, no doubt recalling the Second World War years when Britain had come to the aid of Malta as she fought valiantly against intensive Nazi bombing and suffered a lengthy siege. HM King George VI awarded the island the George Cross for the courage and resilience displayed by the islanders. Emotionally it was a very moving evening and one that made me extremely proud to be British.

We elicited a cornucopia of evidence overall and our Malta police colleagues were pleased to arrest a number of local criminals that had been a constant thorn in their side for more serious offences than usual thanks to our provision of their illegal bank account data. We bade a successful and grateful adieu to Malta and headed for a short stop in Milan in order to clear up some loose ends before finalizing our investigations in Rome. Loose ends cleared up after a couple of days in Milan, we headed to the airport to catch an internal Alitalia flight to Rome. Our hosts escorted us and as we exchanged pleasantries an announcement on the airport tannoy system informed us that our flight, and all others that evening, had been cancelled due to fog. Fog is a common problem at Milan airport, apparently. We'd made appointments with the *Squadra Mobile* in Rome who had detained suspects on our behalf, as well as with the British Embassy to pick up an interpreter, so it was important that we got to Rome early the next day.

To make matters worse, Alitalia couldn't trace our luggage. Fortunately I held all of our important documentation within my in-flight briefcase. Our hosts knew of a night sleeper train to Rome that would get us there in time so they drove us to the relevant railway station and secured us a carriage after an extended conversation with a senior railway orderly. I'm not sure, but I've a sneaking suspicion that some poor travellers were told they had double-booked on their arrival at the station. My Fraud Squad colleague, who it's fair to say liked his grub, set off to buy us a snack for the journey. He returned with fresh bread, olives, cheese, ham and a couple of bottles of a fine Chianti. As our train departed the station and we got comfortable discussing our itinerary in Rome, nibbling away at our tasty snack, there was a knock on the door. A smartly-uniformed orderly entered carrying a tray upon which was what we learned was our supper. This consisted of fresh bread rolls, olives, cheese, ham and a bottle of Italian red wine. London buses, eh!

On being met by the *Squadra Mobile* liaison officer, we received more annoying news to the effect that his counterparts in Milan had informed him that our luggage had been mistakenly flown to Malmo, Sweden. On an internal Italian flight, how does that happen? We were dressed in casual clothes for our train trip but needed to be suited and booted to attend Rome's High Court for the required *commission rogatoire* procedure and follow-up meetings so I contacted Scotland Yard, explained the situation, and was granted authority to spend whatever was required to purchase our clothing requirements. A quick trip to one of Rome's finest gentlemen's clothing establishments saw each of us obtaining an emergency wardrobe so we'd be suitably attired for court. After a hectic day we were dropped off at our hotel, only to find that our luggage had miraculously turned up.

Two days into this aspect of the investigation the newly-appointed pope died, only some thirty-three days after being elected. This time Italy went into lockdown and we again had to spend a couple of days without our escort, again adopting the mantle of tourists. We visited the magnificent Vatican which I recall was packed wall to wall with priests and nuns from all over the world. Once normal service was resumed and we returned to work we completed our investigations and headed home. Another pope was duly elected after a very short selection process and he chose to commemorate his predecessor by taking the name of Pope John Paul II.

Chapter 15

Back to Normal

Yet again a call came into the Bow Street nick to the effect that a woman had been found dead in suspicious circumstances in a bedroom of an extremely well-known hotel in The Strand so I hurried down to seek out the former Glasgow City police DI who I knew was in charge of security there. It transpired that a young woman had been discovered 'trussed up like a chicken', as a young PC who was one of the first officers to attend the scene described his finding of her to me. I summoned the on-call police surgeon to confirm that life was extinct, then alerted my DCI and awaited instructions. Like most of my central London CID colleagues, I knew that many hotels in the West End were aware that prostitutes and escorts used their facilities for business purposes. It appeared from the outset that this lady may be one of that ilk.

Sure enough, the victim was found to be a young woman from the north of England who had used a cheap day British Rail ticket deal to spend a weekend in London working as an escort to earn a bit of cash, not uncommon then, nor, I suspect, even today. The particular rail ticket was advertised as an Away Day deal so the ladies who used them were referred to by local participants in the red light trade as Away Day girls. The pathologist could not ascertain definitely if she died intentionally by another's hand because the nature of her bondage was such that there could have been a consensual element and it may have been that in the throes of passion she inadvertently asphyxiated. What was suspicious was the skedaddling of the occupant of the room who'd left in the wee small hours before her body was discovered. Enquiries to trace him took colleagues to Paris where unfortunately their pursuit ended because he'd flown on to Senegal where there is no extradition treaty with the UK. He will, however, have remained on the Interpol wanted list ever since.

A fellow Bow Street CID officer, who was another native of Fife, and I were tasked to travel to the woman's home town by the DCI, who believe it or not was also a Fifer, to trace and interview friends, family and a host of contacts mentioned in a diary found in the victim's personal belongings. Suffice to say we confirmed that she did work in the sex trade from time to time. We interviewed other women similarly employed who popped down to London to bolster their ailing bank accounts in this manner. One of these women, who knew the victim well, confirmed by the fact that her details were in the victim's diary, confided in us that the main reason that she personally got involved in the sex trade was she just loved having sex. She offered to show us some outfits she wore when entertaining regular clients and enlightened us with the fact that her St Trinian's schoolgirl uniform, as well as her nurse's and WPC outfits were by far the most requested. She even generously offered us a two for the price of one 'totally satisfying session' as she had a thing for coppers. You have to believe me when I tell you that we diplomatically declined her kind offer. She was helpful, however, in relation to background info on the victim.

What we didn't expect were the two men our victim had regularly visited at their home addresses, with the total acquiescence of their spouses who remained present in another room throughout her visits to their respective homes. These couples were not aware of each other's involvement with the deceased, I must stress. In one case the wife was suffering from a debilitating disease and had no libido. The other found the act of intercourse far too painful in which to participate but didn't want her old man to either leave her or be caught kerb-crawling for a street prostitute in seeking some comfort there. Each of these women had contacted the victim and arranged a meeting with her and after a sort of interview requested her to 'see to their respective hubbies' needs'. There were also a few inadequate and lonely men she'd visited regularly because they couldn't communicate with women in the normal way. A tart with a heart, indeed.

A common deception carried out by toms in the West End is known as 'clipping'. In layman's terms it's when a tourist, more often than not a visiting foreign businessman, is approached by a pretty young thing in a pub or hotel where she chats him up, then makes him an offer of her special services which he is not likely to refuse. Once hooked, the punter would be asked for a cash deposit so that she could pop around to a hotel she frequented to ensure it was suitably clean and ready for their use. Believe me, quite a few gullible men fell for this guise and so the girls and their pimps made a lot of money out of it. Most of these punters had expense accounts so they could recover their outlay from the company by other means if they were shrewd enough. Some had no idea of the exchange rate, so blinded by lust, they'd hand over several hundred pounds, or the equivalent, to these ladies who they would never lay eyes on again, surprise, surprise.

A visiting Greek businessman had been caught up in this scam and believe it or not had handed over £400 in cash to a young tom. We knew that these girls would often disappear for a short while and then return, looking for another sucker to dupe. To try to identify the perpetrator, a colleague and I placed the Greek punter in an unmarked CID car and cruised around the Soho streets to see if we could find her as this had proved fruitful in the past. It was early evening and quite warm so we had the car windows down. As we turned a corner we suddenly heard a female voice screaming aloud. We identified roughly where it came from so pulled up and left our victim in the police car with instructions to remain there.

The shrieking continued as we reached a block of flats where a middle-aged woman of Mediterranean appearance stood at the street door looking somewhat distressed. We showed her our warrant cards and she told us that she'd just dialled 999 because a young female resident in the block was obviously being attacked. This lady was a kind of warden and was in possession of a pass key. We ran up a flight of stairs, still with the screams resounding in our ears, where she unlocked the door from behind which the sound obviously came. As we entered we could see that furniture in this small bedsit apartment was in disarray. A young woman was lying face down on a mattress atop a single bed near the window in the opposite wall which she was gripping tightly with both hands. Her knuckles were white with the exertion. Her clothing was partly torn and dishevelled. Lying across her back was a young man with his left arm around her neck trying to prise her off the mattress with his jeans and underpants pulled down to his ankles. He was shouting something unintelligible while she sobbed and screamed.

We grabbed hold of him, noting that his penis was in an erect state. To be frank I think he was initially oblivious to our presence. He reminded me of a dog mounting a bitch in heat that seems to go into a daze. If I'd had a bucket of water, I'd have thrown it over him. After a short but severe struggle he was cuffed and told to calm down. About this time uniform colleagues burst in having responded to the lady warden's 999 call. I asked them to bang him up in a cell at the local nick, ensuring that they removed his clothing for forensic examination, and to let the custody officer know that I'd be there as soon as possible to deal with him. After making sure the female was okay and didn't need hospital treatment, although she had some bruises and scratches on her face and neck, we drove her to the police station where a police surgeon was summoned to record and treat her injuries.

She confirmed that she'd just recently taken up a post in a West End hotel, having travelled from her native Poland seeking employment. Her attacker was a sous-chef in the same establishment. They each had a room in the block where the offence had taken place which was owned by the hotel group. She knew virtually no-one, spoke very little English and had only accepted an invitation to have a drink with the chef after work because he was a workmate and she was a bit lonely. Through an interpreter we established that according to her, the chef attacked her almost immediately they entered his room. She was a devout Catholic and a virgin and gave him no reason to believe she would indulge in any sexual activity. According to him, it was consensual rough sex. I charged him with attempted rape and sexual assault. He was initially remanded in custody, but on a subsequent court appearance was granted conditional bail. For personal security purposes the hotel group agreed the victim's transfer to another of their hotels outside of London away from any contact with her attacker.

At the trial the defence barrister tried all the tricks in his insidious repertoire to clear his man. According to his client, the victim had egged him on, run her hands over his manhood and begun kissing him as soon as they sat on his bed. He didn't know why she'd screamed. The overturned furniture in the room was caused by my colleague and I when we kicked the door in. Of course this was not the case: the door had not been kicked in because the warden had opened it with her pass key. We'd lied about his state of undress and penile erection because we were racists. The defendant was of West Indian origin. The jury took little time in finding him guilty. The learned judge acceded to a request by defence counsel to offer a payment to the victim by way of an apology from his client for the distress his misinterpretation of events had caused her. When I explained this to her via the court interpreter, she became quite distressed and started to cry. She reiterated that she was a virgin and a deeply religious person and that the accused had lied about her. As she saw it, he had just paid for her services as if she were a prostitute. The judge and prosecution counsel were still on the premises so I explained the situation to counsel and asked if the judge would reconsider the defence application. Counsel explained there was no precedent in law for a reversal so the apology and fiscal award were left on file. The victim never claimed it.

This was yet another example of legal counsel twisting events to the detriment of witnesses, especially police officers, for the potential benefit of their client well above and beyond cross-examination and acceptable testing of evidence. It was becoming rare as an active police officer giving evidence in court not to have serious allegations made against you. The sous-chef received a suspended prison sentence, I think because he had not come before a criminal court before. This also disturbed the victim greatly, so much so that she returned to Poland soon afterwards.

Prostitutes were, and hopefully still are, very good police informants if handled properly (no pun intended). They need to be shown respect, and treated decently and protected. In their murky world they regularly brush shoulders with petty and not so petty criminals and could be nurtured into providing police with good sources of criminal activity intelligence. I ran a couple of them as informants while attached to West End police stations with some degree of success.

One night after a very successful conclusion to a difficult investigation a few of us went to a favourite wine bar in the West End to celebrate. Unfortunately this went on much longer than anticipated which ended with a couple of us crashing out in a local hotel room for a few hours before our tour of duty commenced the next day. We made our way to the uncrowned centre of fashion in London then, Carnaby Street in Soho, to buy fresh underwear, socks and a shirt so that we wouldn't look too dishevelled. Spotting a sale on in one of the more popular outlets, there two of us also bought a new suit. Mine was a green corduroy three-piece with flared trousers and brown leather patches on the elbows of the jacket. A dedicated follower of fashion was I. It was a bit loud, I admit, so thereafter I normally wore the trousers with another jacket or the jacket and waistcoat with different trousers. It would seem I had consumed too much alcohol the night before.

A few years later, by which time I'd moved on from the West End, I received a phone call from a DCS at West End Central nick who was investigating a murder. In effect his officers had been approached by a tom who claimed to know pertinent facts about this incident. She told the officers that in the past she'd given good info to a Scots detective at West End Central, adding that occasionally he'd worn a garish green suit. I admitted that it had indeed been me and stressed that she was worth listening to as she'd supplied regular and accurate information to me resulting in several good arrests. I was able to confirm to the guvnor her 'street name' when she was rewarded for her assistance from the Met Police Informants' Fund so that he could verify her credentials.

For my sins I took charge of the Crime Squad for a while. This was fascinating and challenging work. Uniform officers who wished to join the CID were selected to work in plain clothes to see if they had what was required to make this leap. Not all made the grade, of course. Some actually asked to return to uniform duty when they found they were not suited to this aspect of police work or more often because of the long hours we worked and the tedious observations and difficult surveillance operations that had to be carried out before arrests were made. I felt privileged to be part of this selection system and also to watch those I'd help train flourish into substantive detectives, some of whom I'd encounter further along our respective career paths.

On 30 March 1979 Airey Neave, DSO, OBE, MC, the former Shadow Secretary of State for Northern Ireland, was the subject of a fatal explosion in his car as he drove out of the members' car park of the Palace of Westminster. The Irish National Liberation Army (INLA), a banned terrorist organization, had placed a magnetic ball-bearing tilt-switch bomb under his vehicle, causing the loss of both their victim's legs followed by his death shortly afterwards in hospital. Neave had a formidable military record, being one of the few British PoWs to escape from the infamous Nazi prison for Allied officers at Colditz. He also played a lead role in the trials of many Nazi war criminals at Nuremburg after the end of the Second World War. Such a tragic loss.

A memorial service was held on his behalf in May 1979 at St Martin-in-the-Fields Church, Trafalgar Square in central London and my Crime Squad was tasked to assist with security surrounding this venue. Part of the brief was to randomly check the contents of women's handbags as they ascended the steps to attend the function. For this particular task several female members of the team were specifically briefed. Obviously discretion was paramount to security concerns due to the high profile of many of the guests. The rest of us, mere males, were to provide extra eyes and ears to the uniform security detail.

The then Prime Minister Margaret Thatcher arrived with her personal bodyguard as we were carrying out these duties, the female officers occasionally checking ladies' handbags. As the PM ascended the steps, she obviously noticed what was being done so she approached one of the officers, opened her handbag and showed it to her. Once all of the guests were safely inside this fine old church building and the immediate security situation completed, I asked the WPC what she'd seen inside the PM's handbag. To my surprise, she told me that she had no recollection. She was so nervous at being confronted by the PM that she didn't really look into the bag at all. I can't blame her. On the other hand, the naughty side of me wanted to know if perhaps Mrs Thatcher usually carried a tasteful wee hipflask or an elegant ladies' cigarette case around with her.

Like all CID officers in the Met I was transferred every couple of years or so and also attended various courses to enhance my professionalism, gain investigative experience and keep up with ever-changing legislation. I moved from 'C' Division back to 'W' Division and general CID duties, one of which was liaison police officer to HM Prison Wandsworth; not a task popular with CID officers and normally allocated to the new boy on the block, in this case yours truly. Frequent liaison visits with prison security staff for the purposes of investigating drug importation, assaults and weapon recovery plus obtaining any pertinent criminal intelligence on certain inmates were the mainstay of this work, which for obvious reasons nearly always led no further due to lack of witness assistance... surprise, surprise. Prison officers dealt with most of these cases within HMP rules and the prison governor presided as judge and jury.

However, in 1986 an inmate forcibly took hostage a former Rhodesian police officer by the name of Richard Pike, now a prison officer at HMP Wandsworth operating in the hospital wing. The inmate, an extremely violent individual and persistent criminal named Martin Foran, was serving a ten-year sentence as a result of a conviction for a series of armed robberies handed down at Birmingham Crown Court in 1978. A further eight years were added in 1985 for a further robbery charge. Foran maintained his innocence during his incarceration, claiming that West Midland Serious Crime Squad officers had framed him. He'd previously separately undertaken a hunger strike and rooftop protest at other prisons. His family was running a freedom and injustice campaign on his behalf at this time too, but it seems things were not moving fast enough for Foran.

Foran overpowered Officer Pike as the latter attended to one of Foran's medical conditions and held him hostage within a blockaded hospital wing cell for many hours. The door could not be breached due to the fact that in this old Victorian building the hospital wing cell doors opened outwards. Police were called to the scene as well as a specially-trained prison officer intervention team, then me. During the standoff Pike was roughly tied to the bed by his neck and bound. The noose around his neck was frequently yanked by Foran during the siege. While engaged in discussions with negotiators, Foran broke a sample glass into which he threatened to urinate, then cut the officer's throat with it. He claimed to have AIDS and other sexually-transmitted diseases. A pair of scissors was also brandished at the officer's throat. Pike's throat was in fact cut in the assault; fortunately not too seriously, no thanks to the perpetrator.

The conclusion of this hostage-taking, subsequent interviews of Foran plus my investigation into Officer Pike's horrifying ordeal led to Foran being formally charged with a number of serious offences for which he received another six years' imprisonment in the highest court of the land, i.e. the Central Criminal Court at the Old Bailey in 1987.

Officer Pike never returned to active duties as a front-line prison officer. His health suffered, both physically and mentally. As a result he was transferred to a lower category prison in the Birmingham area where he remained until resigning from the prison service on medical grounds. I kept in touch with Richard and his lovely wife Lyn, a nurse, during the period awaiting trial and assisted his application for Criminal Injuries Compensation because of his ongoing medical condition, so I came to know them pretty well. A loving couple who really felt let down by the prison service and their local members of parliament who, in their eyes, were more interested in the campaign to prove Foran's innocence than in their dilemma.

Ironically after twenty-eight years the Court of Appeal upheld Foran's submission for the 1978 convictions which then had a sort of domino effect on the other offences he had committed and of which he was subsequently convicted. Is this the world-renowned British justice of which we're so proud? Not for Richard and Lyn Pike.

Shortly after this incident I had a stint in a sedentary post at New Scotland Yard for eighteen months where I was engaged in researching and screening informants who sought to become what the press called 'Supergrasses'. The Met referred to them as resident informants because once granted this status, they would be taken into protective custody for the duration of their time awaiting trial for their own criminal misdemeanours while supplying witness evidence mainly against fellow armed robbers. Although I found the latter post most interesting, extremely demanding and professionally intriguing and was privileged to be part of this small hand-picked unit through which I became involved with some of the most active, successful and dedicated senior detectives, I still looked forward to returning to front-line investigations again. A successful conclusion of this post saw me looking around for other challenges when out of the blue I was recalled to Flying Squad duties.

To add to this good news I became a dad for a second time in March 1981 when a lovely little daughter who we named Ceri came into our lives. Another reason to be thankful.

Chapter 16

Recalled to Flying Squad Duties

This time I was to be based at the historic Tower Bridge police station assigned to 11 Squad with armed robbery and organized serious and serial crime as our brief. To say the least, this was to become the absolute highlight of my police career. The fantastic chemistry and camaraderie I experienced with this elite band of experienced and dedicated thief-takers happily continues to this day, from guvnors to drivers, in as much as it is the only annual reunion dinner I attend with the guys each November when we catch up, reminisce and generally enjoy a good chat, accompanied by fine food and the odd glass of wine.

Within each Squad officers assist one another all the time in identifying and building a case file on potential criminal targets, and with larger enquiries other Squad team members may be invited to join the show. When such an enquiry starts to really build up, indicating that the criminal may be planning a job, you readily offer assistance whether it be in the OP or obo (observations) van or whatever task is required. It's all part of the special camaraderie mentioned above. In the day-to-day work it's normal to operate as a pair, or as a trio if you're part of a crew of a gunship (fast-response unmarked vehicle containing armed officers). My partner for most of these memorable years in 11 Squad was DS John Pearse [aka JP], a Fulham football club fan but I don't hold that against him. JP is undeniably the most thorough, dedicated and professional partner I ever worked with. He's really bright and a proper nice guy who was also a very good, competent and well-respected detective who thought out of the box more often than not. Our gunship driver was the inimitable Chalky White. Nearly every officer in the Met with the surname of White is nicknamed Chalky, but our Chalky was a bit special and still is, now well into his 80s.

Flying Squad drivers were a unique breed. They were all PCs having attained the highest level of defensive and offensive driving skills that the Met could provide. They were nearly all trained and authorized in the use of firearms as well. However, one of their invaluable and pretty much unknown talents outside of the Squad was their vast knowledge of good greasy spoon cafés and cheap but quality eating places throughout south London which had been gleaned from their years driving uniform patrol cars on division. After early-morning spins it was normally a driver who suggested such a venue. I had the finest devilled kidneys on toast I've ever eaten in one of these cafés, thanks to Chalky.

No matter what length of retention on observations or surveillance, the drivers always claimed an extra thirty minutes at the end of their tour of duty and the same period prior to commencing the next tour. According to them this was in order to carry out 'cockpit drill', their verbal description of checking their high-powered vehicles inside-out to ensure they were up to the high standard required in case of a blues-and-twos call (use of siren and lamps in an emergency). They were required by regulation to park their Squad cars at a police station near to their home address when not in use, but this was mainly ignored because most drivers took their mollycoddled motors home with them. Very occasionally they would use them for unauthorized personal purposes. Chalky fell foul of such a decision once when he had a 'touch' (only slight damage accident) returning from a social occasion and had to call upon the services of an experienced and trusted panel-beating mate to rectify the damage overnight. This set him back a couple of hundred quid; a fact of which he reminded us more than once. To make matters worse, a few weeks later the Met garage responsible for the issue and maintenance of these vehicles contacted Chalky with the news that his beloved 'motor' was to be taken out of service and sold at auction because it had reached the end of its 'shelf life'. Chalky was not amused; after all, he'd just invested a lot of his own cash in the vehicle. He appealed the decision, but the garage won the day.

We'd received a tip-off that an individual who was on our wanted list and probably in possession of a firearm was preparing to commit another armed robbery soon. Chalky drove the Squad car, call sign Central 912, near to the location where our suspect was expected, according to an informant. Another colleague, then a DC, who we shall call 'Eric' for the purposes of this tale and to spare his blushes if he ever reads this missive, accompanied JP and myself. Eric was not yet firearm-trained so his task would be to cuff and search the suspect once we'd disarmed him and

97

made him safe at gunpoint. Like all best-laid plans, when the adrenaline is flowing things don't always go according to plan. Our suspect turned up as expected, so Chalky roared Central 912 towards him and halted. JP and I drew our issued Smith & Wesson revolvers, alighted and, using the nearside doors as cover, knelt down thrusting our firearms in his direction while shouting that we were armed police officers. The suspect started to produce what we identified as a sawn-off shotgun from under his coat as Eric ran directly in front of us, blocking our view and in the direct path of any shots we may have had to take. I was looking at Eric's back a few feet in front of me and now didn't have clear sight of the suspect's hands. A real problem. Bugger. I called out words to the effect that 'If you don't put the gun down right now we will shoot you, even if it means our mate gets injured.' Thankfully he froze with the shotgun still pointing towards the ground and shouted, 'Okay, okay, don't shoot.' We were able to safely remove the weapon, letting Eric cuff him. When the prisoner was banged up and we went for a coffee in the canteen in the local nick, Eric humbly apologized for getting in our way, saying that excitement had got the better of him. He also wanted to know if we would have fired our weapons. I told him I'd tell him at an appropriate time. Eric was nearly retired before I told him that only if the suspect had looked like he was actually going to discharge the shotgun in his direction would I have pulled the trigger. A shotgun, especially one with sawn-off barrels, discharged at that range meant all three of us were in immediate danger of being seriously injured, or even worse, especially Eric.

Tooting and Mitcham areas became 'happy hunting grounds' for 11 Squad. We took out an armed firm about to hit a cash-in-transit bullion van outside Barclays Bank in Upper Tooting Road. The outgoing DI and incoming DI had a little tête-à-tête over who should give the attack order over our radio network from the OP as the bullion van drew up near to where the suspects sat in a stolen vehicle. We burst from our place of concealment anyway and took them down without a shot being fired. A hidden bonus was that this took place outside the branch of a bank where I'd opened a personal account when I first came to London. Naturally after the wannabe blaggers were locked up I returned to the branch in question to help take witness statements from the staff, including the manager. Once I informed this gentleman how much money the Squad had saved his branch that morning, not to mention the potential danger and distress from which we had saved his staff, I thought he might look favourably on any request I might make for an overdraft in the future. If you don't ask, you don't get in this life. Isn't that right?

Not that far away in distance and time another trio turned up in a stolen car as a Post Office bullion van was arriving for a scheduled pick-up quite close to Tooting Police Station situated at Amen Corner. As they pulled on their balaclavas and went to the boot of their car to collect the ubiquitous and much-favoured weapon of choice of blaggers, their sawn-off shotguns, we alighted at speed from our discreetly-parked pantechnicon van and again successfully accomplished a pavement job without injury and without any shots being fired. The only slight hiccup occurred as we exited from the rear of the vehicle at speed, the plan being to turn immediately left out of the rear doors of the van where the blaggers' car sat a few feet away. Most of us did so, but one of our colleagues turned right and was seen by an elderly lady shopper running along the opposite pavement with his handgun held aloft. It took him a few seconds to realize his error. He then ran back towards us, bumped into the lady, apologized and re-entered the fray. We learned of this later when she made a witness statement. Our disorientated colleague subsequently paid his dues at a bar of his choice. Such things can and do happen when the adrenaline, excitement and anticipation levels shoot up immediately before and during an armed operation, no matter what amount of training and planning has been done beforehand.

It's difficult to explain the mixture of feelings that swamps you when awaiting the attack call in these pavement jobs. Often after many weeks of boring, sometimes tedious but necessary surveillance, the anticipation, exhilaration, anxiety and expectation that runs through your head as you check your firearm (for the umpteenth time), secure your flak jacket and mentally run through the detailed attack instructions replaces all other considerations around the impending arrest scenario. When the order is given, the intensive training ordinarily takes over. The rush of testosterone and adrenaline coupled with a greatly increased heart rate flings you towards the armed prey without real consideration of danger (normally). It's similar, I suspect, albeit to a much lesser degree, to paratroopers awaiting the green light to jump from an aircraft. The paramount emotion is, however, fear. Fear that you may let your colleagues down... Fear that you may freeze on hearing the attack call… Fear of being shot…and – rather bizarrely you may think – fear of having to discharge your weapon and perhaps take the life of another human being.

In those days Flying Squad officers were lightly-armed with Smith & Wesson six-shot revolvers, either Model 10 or the snub-nose Detective's Special Model 12, the latter being lighter and easier to conceal. Neither was particularly accurate except at close range, which is where you didn't really want to be if at all possible because most often we would face criminals armed with sawn-off shotguns and a variety of handguns often more powerful than our issued revolvers. Firearms training was basic and only conducted four times a year. We relied on the bad guys losing their bottle or not knowing if their weapons would actually work, coupled with their misconception that we were highly trained and motivated. Thankfully this combination normally paid off.

The whole process is usually all over in a few minutes and is recorded on video by a designated colleague so that no allegations of fitting up or planting weapons can be made at a later date, but more importantly so that the court can see exactly what happened and who was in possession of what at the time of the arrest. It's also often a boon during the interviewing process when the accused can be shown the video and realize that he's bang to rights and caught red-handed. The buzz of satisfaction of a good job well done permeates the transportation to the designated police station where the guvnor will select the interview teams while other team members return to the scene to take statements from any witnesses or victims as appropriate and supervise photographing in detail the location and any weapons contained there which will be retrieved and packaged in accordance with evidence-handling procedures. Other officers will be tasked to execute search warrants at the known homes of the arrested persons where often others will be arrested for conspiracy to commit armed robbery or kindred offences. It's a complex time but one conducted regularly and extremely professionally by the Sweeney.

On another occasion JP and I were trying to trace an individual wanted for armed robbery utilizing JP's old Renault car for surveillance purposes. He had a few old bangers during our stint together, did JP. Our suspect walked by so we rushed out and cuffed him after a bit of a struggle. As JP leaned into his car to summon a uniform van via radio and I held onto the prisoner, the latter said: 'Are you sure you guys are the Sweeney? I mean, that's a really crap motor.' I don't think JP was amused. Another investigation found us both pushing shopping trolleys around a south London supermarket that we suspected was about to be robbed, each of us separately adopting the role of bona fide shoppers with our 'other halves' being female surveillance officers alongside us. The arrest team waited in the security office watching through a one-way glass screen. According to them, we looked the business. We did this over several weekends before others in the team nicked the suspected crew sitting in a motor outside the premises with the usual paraphernalia and charged them with conspiracy to commit armed robbery and kindred firearm offences. Thank goodness. I don't like shopping at the best of times, but pretend shopping is even worse.

When not involved in actual surveillance or research of target criminals, we responded to all armed robberies in the south London area which were broadcast on our radio network in order to assist local divisional detectives. On one such occurrence a middle-aged black male walked into a bank in Queenstown Road, Battersea armed with a sawn-off shotgun and demanded the cash contents of the tills. He barked at the few customers present, ordering them to place their hands on their heads and get down on the floor, which most of them did apart from a middle-aged gent who remained standing. Our gallant robber went over to him, pressed the ends of the shotgun barrels into his face, and again demanded that he get down on his knees. The gent remained standing with his hands aloft and refused to kneel. The robber shoved him up against the wall, repeatedly shouting 'Don't move, don't move' as he grabbed a couple of money bags that the cashiers had filled with cash. He then backed out of the premises 'Bonnie and Clyde style' while covering everyone with his shotgun.

Unfortunately for him the much younger getaway driver who should have been waiting for him in a nicked car had bottled it, probably at the sound of a passing police siren, so was nowhere to be seen. Our robber then ran towards Battersea Dogs Home and into a petrol station where he was seen by staff dumping stuff in a litter bin and running off. When they checked the bin they found a shotgun wrapped in an anorak. Our man then entered a mini-cab firm and tried to muster a cab. It was a busy time of day so there would be quite some delay which he obviously didn't fancy so again he ran off. Staff noticed that he was in an agitated state and they would later tell detectives he carried what looked like a couple of bank cash bags with the bank's logo showing stuffed down his trousers but partly protruding at the belt.

It became obvious that our man was probably local and not very good at his chosen career. Enquiries made of the local nicks threw up a suspect, so we began digging around to trace him. A couple of known former addresses were visited by colleagues and the occupants spoken to. A former girlfriend was traced and although she was willing to assist due to the domestic violence she'd received at his hands when they were together, she was not really up to date on his whereabouts. However, as luck would have it an observant PC had seen our man a few days beforehand entering a local address and he thankfully recorded the fact. Coupled with this info a DC on our team who'd served as a local CID officer in the area received a tip-off from an informant corroborating that this was our man and confirmed he used this address.

Colleagues keeping watch on the house established his presence so we carried out a 'hard entry' and he was arrested. A search of the address once he and his latest lady friend had quietened down revealed a couple of bank cash bags and a few grand in notes. Both were taken to the local nick where he maintained his innocence throughout the interviews, alleging that we had brought the bags with us 'to fit him up'.

Because he possessed a previous conviction for armed robbery and many others for serious and major crime he was remanded in custody at his initial appearances before local magistrates. In those days it was virtually impossible to get male members of the black community to assist police with identity (ID) parades. The black community simply didn't trust the police. No matter what fees or reassurances were offered, such a request fell upon deaf ears so because of this Brixton police officers had come up with an excellent compromise which was acceptable in the courts.

A suspect who agreed to an ID parade was detained by uniform colleagues on a platform on the underground system where he was allowed to join passengers at his discretion as they disembarked from any train and ascended the escalator to the ground-level exit. At the exit point to the street other uniform officers would cause the relevant witnesses to step forward and indicate if he or she saw the suspect for their particular crime. The uniform inspector in charge briefed the witnesses that if they felt they could, they should touch anyone they had seen committing the crime on the shoulder or, if unable to do this, to point that person out to him. We decided to use this method to conduct an ID for the Queenstown Road armed robbery. Accordingly our suspect's legal representative was present as were JP and I, but simply as observers. Procedure forbade us taking an active part. We were present simply to witness the event.

Our suspect chose the train and his position on the escalator as described and as he reached the top the middle-aged gent who had defied the robber's barked demands during the robbery walked briskly up to him and prodded him roughly on the chest, saying words to the effect that 'That's the bastard.' The inspector noted this as a positive identification. The suspect's legal representative made a half-hearted protest while noting details on her clipboard. All were taken to the local nick where a further witness statement was taken from this witness. It transpired that he'd been a former British army soldier who'd seen active service in Korea. His courage had not diminished with time, it would appear.

Meanwhile, the bank staff who didn't wish to attend an ID parade had attended Witness Albums at Scotland Yard. Here they were shown photograph albums of suspects who had been convicted of such crimes and who fitted the witness's description. Sadly none of them picked our man out. This is not unusual because in such circumstances most individuals do not look directly at the suspect's face, especially one brandishing a sawn-off shotgun in their general direction. This is known as weapon focus effect and is well documented in scientific journals.

The suspect maintained his innocence during the trial, clinging to his allegations of Flying Squad corruption and evidence-planting. His defence team maintained that some of the civilian witnesses were lying because of duress from Flying Squad officers as well as others simply being mistaken and, for the final throw of the defence dice, that they were racists. The jury took no little time in deliberating on all the contested evidence in this case, but eventually saw through this subterfuge and the man was convicted. Sentencing him for a lengthy period, the learned judge commended the Flying Squad investigation team for their professionalism and detective ability and, appropriately, the former soldier for his personal courage. He had impressed the judge due to his detailed recall of the weapon carried by the robber and also his accurate description of the man's facial features.

I'll never understand why our hapless but nevertheless dangerous robber didn't cover up his face. During questioning we noted he displayed a habit of slightly but frequently flicking his tongue lizard-like in and out between his lips when he displayed the characteristics of becoming obviously nervous. This activity was recorded in one of our interviews by our guvnor DI Grieve who incidentally was researching body language and related matters while studying for a psychology degree at the time. During the trial he was able to assist the court with his observations as he informed the judge and jury how the suspect reacted to specific questions put to him by JP and I. A first for all of us. Obviously this was vigorously contested by the defence.

The suspect was doing this as he rode the escalator during the ID parade and the former soldier recalled this exact same behaviour when the guy was barking out demands in the bank on the day. No doubt he had plenty of time to reflect upon this blunder as he served his lengthy prison sentence. By way of closure and to dispel the myth that honour among thieves exists, if my memory serves me well his girlfriend proffered the identity of the getaway driver in order that she would not be charged with any serious criminal offence.

It is not just a coincidence that later on in their respective impressive years as Scotland Yard detectives Messrs Grieve (JG) and Pearse (JP) combined their many talents and expertise in psychology, especially effective interrogation techniques, in compiling a first-class book well respected within the world of forensic psychology as it relates to terrorist investigations. By this time JP had studiously obtained a few impressive letters behind his name, viz PhD, CPsychol and AFBPsS. His interest in police interrogative techniques deepened after a criminal trial in which we were both engaged that was brought about by the arrest of a number of men who attempted to rob a bullion van delivery courier of cash meant for the payment of staff wages within a north London hospital. Psychological defects of at least one of the robbers caught in the act was put forward by the defence to good effect (from their point of view, that is) when he was acquitted after the jury found him not guilty. Since retiring from the Met, JP has travelled around the world providing counter-terrorist advice and training through seminars to much well-deserved acclaim. I've alluded to the numerous and varied achievements of JG in another chapter. This period was undoubtedly the pinnacle of my police career in having the opportunity and privilege of working in a remarkable Flying Squad team, especially with these two illustrious colleagues.

The book in question is entitled *Investigating Terrorism: Current Political, Legal and Psychological Issues* and was first published in

2015 by Wiley Blackwell. It's well worth a read for those still involved in counter-terrorism, especially those engaged in the most demanding of interviews of those suspected of involvement in terrorist crimes.

I should probably explain what I meant earlier in this chapter when I referred to a 'hard entry'. To the uninitiated this appears to be a simple kick-door-down exercise followed by rushing in shouting to hopefully bag the suspect before he can cause any injury to anyone or escape. This is what it looks like in fairness, but behind the scenes and in order for the procedure to be successful a lot more is involved. Once the address of the suspect is identified, surveillance will follow. While this is being taken care of, colleagues will check local and national records to build up a picture of the nature of the suspect and in effect conduct a risk assessment for armed entry. It may be decided that this is too dangerous so it would be better to keep eyeball on the premises and have an arrest team secreted nearby to effect an arrest when a suspect leaves the premises.

If, however, it all comes together for a hard entry to be carried out, then those involved will be briefed in detail once an officer of suitable rank – it was a Supt in my day – gives authority for firearms to be issued. Those authorized would draw the weapons from the armoury, then methodically check them and load accordingly. The weapons would then be holstered, with safety catches on. Drivers tended to prefer a holster that was basically pushed into the groin area so that they were relatively comfortable while driving but able to draw the weapon quickly if or when required. Others felt comfortable with a high-rise belt holster that afforded quick access. I preferred a shoulder holster as it was more comfortable to wear and I obtained one from an FBI colleague that could be worn under a shirt in summer when high-rise wearers had to keep their jackets on.

Having been thoroughly trained in the use and carriage of firearms it became almost habitual when authorized to carry one. I must admit that after I was initially authorized I looked forward to an opportunity to prove that I could and would use it if confronted and circumstances demanded. However, after the passage of time with regular carriage the firearm just becomes another piece of kit you carry to do your job. Without you really being aware of it, the regular range training allows training staff to continually assess your psychological capability to carry a lethal weapon as much as your ability to use it. Having said that, it

105

still gave me a buzz as I strapped one on. Overall though, as I think I've covered in several previous examples, the paramount consideration was that it is still, and should remain, a last resort remedy.

The relevant layout of the building in question would be scrutinized as the entry team decided on their separate roles. Drivers normally would be positioned to cover the rear of the premises in case of an escape bid and the key man, who would smash in the front door, would normally volunteer for this task. In 11 Squad we had DC Jack Kelly, nicknamed Wookie because of his alleged resemblance to the *Star Wars* character. He had longish red hair and a kindred beard. One tough cookie was Jack, who really liked 'doing the doors'. On one occasion when he had a bit of trouble effecting entry and eventually fell to the floor over the door he'd just demolished, we literally ran up and over his back to get upstairs and effect an arrest as he lay stock still. He didn't complain too much. That's how it goes and that was classic Jack, our very own key man.

We nearly always briefed a standby gunship crew to form an outside or second cordon in case anyone made a break or a getaway driver tried to evade arrest. We'd learned this from bitter experience and it paid dividends on more than one occasion. We were not an elite unit for nothing.

I always preferred to be in the entry team. I felt a thrill in the actual laying on of hands as we arrested our quarry and the subsequent satisfaction in searching for and finding vital evidence. It was stimulating. As I've alluded to earlier, this usually meant I could also get involved with interviewing the suspects. The battle of minds between a suspect and the detective can be pretty unique, a bit like the thrust and parry between the detective and defence counsel in court at a later stage. I lapped it up, as did most of my peers.

Chapter 17

Blags 'r' Us

A number of armed robberies had already been carried out on licensed betting shops in Kent resulting in Regional Crime Squad (RCS) officers working alongside local detectives trying hard to solve them. They had identified a pattern indicating that the gang responsible might try similar premises in south London soon. This, of course, was 11 Squad's manor. After consultations with RCS colleagues, delving into the criminal intelligence sources at the Yard and rubbing shoulders with some of our own informants, we began to form a profile and were soon able to mount a covert surveillance on the main suspect, which proved fruitful. We observed him and one other take a casual drive-by-style look at a betting shop in Pimlico in south London so we heightened our efforts accordingly. Suffice to say that on a given day we set up an armed ambush so that we could arrest them in the act of armed robbery at this location, or in Squad parlance, 'take them out on the pavement'.

Foot surveillance officers tailed them to the door. We were aware that they were in possession of sawn-off shotguns and masks in a holdall carried by one of them. When they entered the bookmakers' premises a surveillance officer was to literally stick a foot in the door and the arrest team, of which I was one, would immediately spring from our hiding-place and nick them. However, as with all best-laid plans, when they actually did stroll in, the foot surveillance officer had not been able to get close enough to prevent the street door being closed so reported this unfortunate circumstance via her covert radio, adding that the street door had in fact been locked by the last guy in.

We were secreted right next door so when the attack order from the guvnor in an observation post opposite resounded in our ears we ran out onto the pavement. The front of the bookies featured a large opaque window with sporting scenes depicted on it behind which we could hear shouting coming from within. It was common practice during these 'pavement jobs' for some Squad officers to carry wooden staves as well as their firearms. These are similar to those issued to mounted branch officers and would be used against violent but unarmed suspects, some of whom carried (and used) pickaxe handles in their pursuit of crime. I was armed and carrying a stave on this occasion which I decided to use immediately. I smashed it into the window which shattered into very small glass fragments and fell like rain to reveal a robber just inside a few feet from my partner and me with his back to the window. He was holding a sawn-off shotgun. Two other robbers were pointing their weapons at the counter staff on the other side of the shop.

Other members of the arrest team smashed in the street door and, with weapons drawn, entered shouting 'Armed police, armed police, put down your weapons.' The guy standing directly in front of us started to turn around, bringing his weapon pointing towards us. My partner repeated the command 'Armed police, put your weapon down', but I decided what to do before he did and struck him hard in the middle of his forehead with the butt of my stave. He immediately crashed to the floor, so we leaped in, grabbed the shotgun off him and held him face down with his arms behind his back in order to place the cuffs on his wrists. A similar fate befell his partners in crime, minus the use of a stave. No shots were fired and no-one else was injured.

They were all bundled into separate Squad cars and taken to local nicks. Our man's eyes were swelling up rapidly and beginning to close by this time and a very large bump was protruding from his forehead. As soon as we got him into the custody suite I asked that a police surgeon be summoned to inspect his injury. A very youthful uniform duty officer appeared (he looked about 18) to deal with our prisoners and he immediately asked how our man received his injury. I produced my stave, which would be retained as evidence, and briefed him. He looked quite shocked and later admitted he wasn't aware that the Squad used staves. After the police surgeon deemed our man 'fit to be detained' he was interviewed at length, as were his accomplices, then all were charged with attempted robbery and illegal possession of firearms. As I walked him back to his cell he extended his open hand and said: 'I'd like to thank you for not shooting me.' We shook on it. A good day's work indeed. Time, as some in the military used to say, 'to head home for tea and medals'.

Later when one of my colleagues was noting a witness statement from one of the bookmaker's counter staff, he mentioned with a laugh:

'I couldn't believe it when you guys burst in. I thought, surely not two robberies on the same day.' Again the Squad arrest team was appropriately commended for bravery, determination and detective ability by the Crown Court Judge who, when sentencing the robber I'd struck, rather embarrassingly singled me out by saying: 'You are only alive because of the courage of DS Turnbull in not shooting you. He would have been fully justified in doing so.' It's the only time I'm aware of an officer being commended for not doing something. The Met Commissioner echoed his appreciation when he later awarded a few of us his highest commendation to boot.

I carried a covert firearm when necessary over a period of some fifteen years and, like the majority of my police colleagues, am pleased to say that I never fired a shot in anger. I discharged quite a few at various levels of firearm training and drew the weapon a handful of times when effecting an arrest or covering a suspect believed to be armed during search procedures. I've no doubt readers will be aware that the reason armed police officers shout commands at a suspected armed criminal is not just a legal requirement but that the shock, disbelief, loud voices and swift aggressive movements of the officers are intended to disorientate the individual and buy the officers time to disarm and apprehend the suspect without having to pull the trigger. Thankfully in the UK this procedure is normally successful. Not all armed robbery enquiries end up with heroic pavement arrests. Most reach conclusion after a lot of good old-fashioned sleuthing, gumshoeing and painstakingly tedious detective work, as the following two examples bear witness.

A number of armed robberies had occurred in and around the Croydon area occasioned by a lone white male dressed in what was described as an ex-RAF greatcoat. He targeted off-licence premises and late-night petrol stations brandishing a handgun and on one occasion was seen to make his getaway on a pedal cycle. My team was instructed to take a look at these incidents, although they didn't come under Squad guidelines entirely. An officer who had been stationed in the region for a long time put forward the opinion that the circulated photo-fit likeness of the suspect looked like a former T/DC who had resigned from the force to take up security work with a pop group. I recalled the individual from a brief spell when I had been assigned to Croydon nick. As I recall he'd given up a promising police career to travel with this group of musicians as a roadie and security adviser after forming a relationship with one of the female singers.

Delving through local data and chatting with some of his former police colleagues led us to believe that he had indeed travelled extensively with the group, but had eventually returned to the local area several months earlier with the ex-singer and their two young children when the band fell on hard times and broke up. He was now drawing state benefits and apparently living in substandard rented accommodation. We quickly carried out an early-morning raid which found him in squalid conditions and it was obvious that he and his lady friend were habitual drug-users. An ex-RAF greatcoat was found in the flat and there was a bicycle in the hall. He recognized me and agreed to make a statement, insisting that his wife had no knowledge of his misdeeds. He was taken to the local nick where after a lengthy interview he admitted his involvement in these robberies. He was adamant that the handgun was a facsimile and not capable of discharging a bullet. I convinced him the return of the weapon would prove this assertion and probably help his case in the eyes of the court. Thankfully he took this course and we recovered it. It was indeed a fake. It was obvious that drugs had driven him to these desperate measures. As anticipated, the court did take into cognizance his admissions and the recovery of the replica fake weapon plus his social and mental state, especially his drug dependency, but he still received a custodial prison sentence, albeit shorter than it could have been. Such a pointless and sad waste of life for all concerned.

Another south London nick had received a couple of phone calls from an anonymous source implicating a young man who resided locally in an armed robbery. Details given by this source matched an armed robbery committed shortly beforehand in a small village bank branch situated nearby. This also fell on my desk so we started to take a look at it. Before long another phone call came in to local police to the effect that the youth was planning another armed robbery, and soon. This time the source provided an address. On the following Saturday morning we set up an observation vehicle to view the address and I went to the local nick to run searches on it. To my astonishment it was recorded as currently occupied by a recently-retired uniform police sergeant who had been stationed at this very police station and who now operated a driving school from the premises. He resided there with his wife, son and mother-in-law. We returned to the premises and joined the obo van crew. It didn't feel right, so we discussed the situation and after a while decided to knock on the door and take it from there. If it was a hoax or a malicious or vindictive call it could be written off straight away.

The obo van crew covered our backs, just in case, as we knocked on the door which was answered by a lady who we assumed would be the mother-in-law. We showed her our warrant cards and asked for the retired sergeant, only to be told he was out. We therefore asked for the son by name and the lady told us he was up in his room, indicating a room at the top of the stairs. 'Just go up' she said, and straight away walked back into the room from whence she'd come. We took the stairs, knocked on the door and stepped inside to find a young man who fitted the description of the alleged bank robber sitting on a settee reading a magazine. We produced our warrant cards and identified ourselves as Flying Squad officers, only to note his immediate change in demeanour. As my colleague spoke with this now apparently quite nervous individual basically informing him of the reason for our visit, I noticed the handles of a holdall protruding from under the side of the settee on which he was sitting. He saw me looking at it and became even more agitated so I pulled it out, avoiding the handles, asking 'What's this then?' Before he answered, and to my utter disbelief, I could see the outline of what I believed to be a sawn-off shotgun just beneath the partially open zipped top. Neither of us was armed at this time. Note to self: do not let yourself get into this position again!

My colleague on this occasion was fellow DS Chris Buckell; another great guy and first-class detective. Chris asked him a few more detailed questions, then the young man just stood up, placed both arms out in front of him in a stance which invited us to place handcuffs on his wrists, and then broke down in tears. I had a quick look inside the holdall and saw several bundles of banknotes, still with bank tape around them, plus a balaclava and some gloves. We cautioned and arrested the lad and, after leaving one of our colleagues to protect this room for forensic examination and a more thorough search as it was now a crime scene, took him to another local nick where a thorough forensic check of the holdall revealed there were no cartridges in the shotgun. The tape around the banknotes bore the relevant bank address and amazingly even the date of the robbery. Subsequent examination confirmed that they were from the nearby branch robbed earlier. The culprit later led us to a stolen car he had stashed close to his home and had fitted with false plates in which to carry out his next crime.

The story unfolded that he had committed the armed robbery alone (as we suspected), and because he thought it was easy money with minimal risk of being arrested he was preparing to commit another similar offence. Here was yet another young person ruining his life because of drug dependency. One of the more awkward and difficult aspects of this case was breaking the bad news to his parents. His father was aware of the lad's drug abuse, but had no idea how serious his dependency had become. The whole family was devastated. Our guvnor was initially in a state of disbelief, nay denial, when I phoned to tell him that we'd cleared up a blag, arrested the perpetrator, recovered a fair portion of the cash taken, recovered the weapon used in a 'happy bag' and traced a stolen motor vehicle false-plated for use on another similar crime. This was mainly due to the fact that 11 Squad's overtime budget was about to take a bit of a hit as we processed the prisoner, recorded his written admissions and then set up a weekend magistrates court to remand him in custody. Justice doesn't come cheap, believe me.

Chapter 18

Life after the Flying Squad

To say the least I would've been more than happy to remain as a Flying Squad officer for the rest of my police service but that's not how it works. A regular turnover of fresh minds, experience and dedicated detectives is necessary, which makes this unique crime-busting unit the great success it has been over many years. Many countries have tried to emulate the Flying Squad but few get close. I recall a visiting FBI agent telling me that they had law enforcement units as good, if not better, in the USA. I'm aware that the resources of the FBI are second to none, but the calibre of detective is what really counts at the end of the day. At that same function another US law enforcement officer who'd overheard his FBI colleague's comment whispered to me 'Do you know what FBI stands for in the States, Ron?' quickly followed by 'Famous but Incompetent.' Made me laugh. Now you know too.

One of Scotland Yard's assistant commissioners returned from an exchange sabbatical in the USA with a cartload of fresh ideas and law enforcement initiatives that had impressed him. He debriefed the commissioner with those he thought would benefit the Met and probably the entire British police service. He'd been particularly impressed with the highly successful Crimestoppers project which operated in nearly every US State. The then commissioner, the late great Sir Peter Imbert, QPM, decided to install such a system in the Met so, along with vital co-operation from TV and radio channels plus initial funding by ADT, a large security business, it was soon launched. For those readers unaware of Crimestoppers, it's a scheme whereby details of particular crimes are broadcast via television, radio and other media appeals to the public who are requested to contact the team on a dedicated freefone telephone number (0800 555111) if they have any information that may lead to the arrest of the perpetrator/s and/or recovery of stolen goods. A reward may be offered for this info in certain cases. All of the information passed on in this way is dealt with under complete confidentiality.

Led by DI Bill Gent with whom I had worked on many surveillance operations against professional and persistent criminals while a Flying Squad officer, with myself as office manager plus three DCs selected for this unique role and a first-class civilian administrator, we set up our equipment in a small secure office in Scotland Yard that was often visited by the commissioner in person as he kept a close personal eye on our progress. It was his baby, after all. My task, apart from daily management of the team, was to ensure that all information received got to the appropriate investigators in the shortest possible time as well as nurturing these sources into giving more information; in short, recruiting them as informants where possible. Bill and I, accompanied by a representative of the trust formed to drive this project, namely Community Action Trust (CAT), toured the UK giving presentations to many police forces and appeared on local TV and radio promoting same which was extremely interesting. The main questions set before us were with regard to the cash rewards offered to entice information from the general public. Ironically an extremely small number of callers even mentioned a reward but were compelled to pass on their information gratis as a public service. Crimestoppers was a great success, resulting in a large number of arrests and several million pounds worth of stolen property recovered within the first two years of operation. As envisaged, the project is now in use in every UK police force and continues to be a resounding success and another very important tool in a detective's toolbox.

Chapter 19

Laboratory Liaison Officer

During the many criminal trials in which I'd been involved throughout my CID career spanning twenty years at that time, and many others that I hadn't, it was becoming clear that police testimony was being undermined and inappropriately challenged more and more, thus convictions were being lost. Guilty perpetrators were getting off scot free, which was not good for justice or our society, which in my opinion still maintains a legal and policing system the envy of the rest of the civilized world. To enhance my skills and become more involved in evidence corroboration I sought out training courses in forensic investigation, criminology and offender profiling in which tutors from various disciplines, mainly pathology and anthropology, instilled an overall and lasting basis of forensic knowledge in me which I hopefully put to good use over the ensuing years dealing with high-profile murders and terrorist atrocities in London and beyond.

One of the main influences in my turning into a forensic detective was an anthropology and offender profiling course I attended at Ninewells Hospital, Dundee, Scotland. Here Dr Sue Black, OBE, now deservedly a Professor and Dame Commander, the latter being awarded in HM the Queen's Birthday Honours List in 2018, eventually managed to instil a basis of anthropology knowledge in me while other tutors, including former FBI Special Agent Robert Ressler, one of the original FBI agents who set up the Behavioral Science Unit (Criminal Profiling) at the FBI Academy in Quantico, USA, added other intrigues of a forensic and pathology nature. Ressler's team interviewed some of America's most prolific serial killers such as Ted Bundy, John Wayne Gacy ('the killer clown') and David Berkowitz (New York's 'Son of Sam') et al. He conducted a series of lectures on behalf of Michigan State University and I managed to attain a basic certificate in Criminal Profiling. Another first for a Met LLO, by the way.

These factors and individuals led me in 1990 to successfully apply for a position as a Laboratory Liaison Officer (LLO aka Homicide Advisor) at the Metropolitan Police Forensic Science Laboratory (MPFSL) in Vauxhall, south London. The post of LLO was created expressly for career detectives to be trained in advanced forensic recovery methods in order to attend any suspicious death discovered by uniform colleagues and, with this extensive training coupled with their already inbuilt detective ability and experience, make an assessment as to whether the death was suspicious or not, thus saving senior CID officers from being (sometimes needlessly) called out to each body found, which had been the norm for too many years. If the LLO considered the incident to be suspicious he then would take over responsibility for the crime scene examination and commence the process of crime scene awareness, containment and controlled evidence recovery. The LLO had authority to call out police photographers, fingerprint officers, SOCO, pathologists and any scientific discipline within MPFSL or any other forensic experts for that matter that were deemed necessary at these varied and often difficult crime scenes to ensure best practice from the start. This removed the burden from SIOs, many of whom after the LLO system began would not attend a crime scene until the LLO had been informed and was en route, while certain other SIOs wouldn't attend until the LLO had done so and verified the nature of the alleged crime.

In England and Wales the coroner may take an interest in any body lying within his or her jurisdiction, whether referred or not. However, most cases are referred to the coroner by doctors, police and members of the public. Deaths may also be referred by the Registrar of Deaths if a death certificate issued by a doctor is unacceptable, which it may be for the following reasons:

- The deceased was not attended in his/her last illness by the doctor completing the certificate
- The deceased had not been seen by a doctor either after death or within fourteen days prior to death
- Where the cause of death is unknown
- Where death appears to be due to poisoning or to industrial disease
- Where death may have been unnatural or may have been caused by violence, neglect or abortion or where it is associated with suspicious circumstances
- Where death occurred during a surgical operation or before recovery from an anaesthetic.

Once a death is reported the coroner, if he or she is satisfied that it is due to natural causes, can decide not to pursue any further enquiries and request that the doctor issue a death certificate. Alternatively, and more commonly, he or she may order a post-mortem examination (now referred to more frequently by the American term autopsy; colloquially referred to by pathologists, police officers and kindred professionals as a 'special'). Forgive me if I still use the term 'post mortem' as I prefer it. In a similar vein I still prefer the word 'murder' to 'homicide' as used in America which has also crept into common usage here. Call me old-fashioned.

Once designated a suspicious death, the LLO would alert the on-call area CID SIO who would immediately set up a murder investigation team (MIT) to deal with the incident. To say the least, this post required a great deal of responsibility and dedication but was a wonderful opportunity and challenge to those officers who relished involvement in major crime investigation. Under the leadership of a DI, the twelve selected DSs were responsible for the entire Met area split into four regions. I was responsible with two other LLOs for twenty-four-hour cover of south-east London from a site office in Shooters Hill police station, SE18. It's now a block of luxury flats like a great many other former Met buildings, sadly.

We shared an office at MPFSL as well with the remainder of our department who similarly covered the rest of the Met from where we operated a rota system so that when 'on call' we carried our murder kit and consumable forensic packaging in our nondescript vehicles. Initially we were alerted by pager, then were ultimately issued with mobile phones which made getting to the scene and calling out assistance so much more efficient and easier. At the time we thought pagers were at the cutting edge of communication technology but compared to the range of possibilities via smart phones nowadays, they were the equivalent of speaking into tin cans joined together by a very long piece of string. Apart from crime scene work, we attended all relevant post-mortem examinations, thus building up a unique relationship with Home Office forensic pathologists. We took on an area training role as well, ensuring that probationer PCs and later on senior officers who transferred into the CID having not undergone a CID course so that they were up to date with crime scene awareness and ever-changing forensic procedures.

My forensics mentor who became a really good friend was DS Cliff Smith who'd operated in the role for several years prior to me joining the team. Cliff and I went on to work together in UN war crime investigations in the Balkans after retirement from the Met. I attended several call-outs with Cliff taking the lead role until it was jointly agreed that I could go solo. On my first solo attendance I was understandably extremely nervous so I arrived really early and parked up a street or so away from the actual crime scene, then skimmed through my notes to make sure I wouldn't miss anything or fail to call out the appropriate assistance. Of course I needn't have worried because when the LLO (more commonly referred to by police officers as simply the 'Lab Sgt') turns up you can almost feel everyone taking a step backwards because they know it's up to the Lab Sgt from then on in. Gradually working through crime scene after crime scene, your experience grows, your reputation and credibility also grow and SIOs and certain pathologists increasingly rely on your professional opinion and assistance. When an AMIT (Area Major Incident Team) arrives, if circumstances require, an exhibit officer is designated and he or she under the Lab Sgt's direction then records, collects, packages and prepares any exhibits and then compiles any detailed submission forms for onward transmission to the laboratory for any forensic examination that may be required.

One of the most difficult aspects of being a Lab Liaison Officer was attending special post-mortem examinations on a regular basis. Initially it seemed somewhat macabre being present and suitably gowned and masked while the pathologist opened up a cadaver and removed certain vital organs and explored the entire body to recover any evidence of foul play. The nature of this aspect of the role is not for everyone but I soon found these procedures fascinating and, as time went by, I learned a great deal from the experienced pathologists with whom I worked. Many of them were only too happy to pass on valuable tips and advice to a raw LLO, especially in relation to the interpretation of multiple injuries and the description in their professional opinion of the weapon used drawn from detailed examination and measurement of the relevant wound.

The main reasons for conducting an autopsy (to use the conventional description) in the UK are:

- To assist with identification of the body
- To estimate the time of death
- To identify and document the nature and number of injuries
- To interpret the significance and effect of the injuries

- To identify the presence of any natural disease
- To interpret the significance and effect of the natural disease where present
- To identify the presence of poisons
- To interpret the effect of any medical or surgical treatment.

Noting in detail any physical anomalies, tattoos and old injuries present on the body was also essential for identification purposes. Relevant body samples, obviously depending on the nature of the suspicious death, were removed by the pathologist and packaged by the LLO for eventual submission to the laboratory for various analytic examinations. This could include nail clippings, urine samples, stomach contents, bullet fragments and broken-off ends of knives as well as internal and external swabs in cases involving rape or sexual violence. I soon became quite adept at identifying the telltale signs of manual strangulation such as the existence of petechial haemorrhaging in the eyeballs and sometimes a damaged hyoid bone in the larynx, as well as the distinct cherry-pink hypostasis caused by carbon monoxide poisoning, a common method of suicide in which a pipe is led from the exhaust pipe of a motor car into the interior and the engine left running until the person becomes unconscious followed by death from inhalation of these toxic fumes.

Shortly after I went 'live and solo' I was called to a suspicious death in Greenwich, south London. It was just before the rush hour when apparently a male had set fire to himself in his car after having a dispute with his estranged wife who lived nearby. The position of the vehicle was seriously impeding traffic. I lived not far away, so after calling out a photographer and pathologist (to declare life extinct; a legal requirement), I made haste to the scene. When I arrived uniform police were conducting traffic and the fire brigade had corralled their vehicles around the deceased's car which was covered in tarpaulin out of respect for the body within and to protect it from the rain. It was raining heavily and was quite windy so the fire brigade had weighted the tarp down with sandbags. After a short briefing and the arrival of the photographer, I decided to obtain some external photo shots of the vehicle so I pulled back the tarp and could see the occupant within displaying extreme facial, head, arm and upper body burns and he was obviously dead. I bent down to shift a sandbag and nearly did my back in by not anticipating how heavy it was. I think I may have let out a grunt or something similar. At this a female fire-fighter stepped forward saying 'Let me do that sir, we're trained to lift heavy weights', and with obvious ease she moved it away. Sheepishly I thanked her, while inwardly feeling a bit of a wimp. The deceased, it seemed, had turned up outside his estranged wife's address several times before and threatened to kill himself, but after a verbal exchange he usually drove off. On this occasion, however, he'd poured petrol over himself, telling her over his mobile phone what he was doing, then lit his cigarette lighter and the rest is history. Fire Investigation Unit (FIU) scientists from MPFSL confirmed this, as did the pathologist at the post-mortem examination.

Fire, in terms of arson, has been used for centuries to cover up crime, so when attending such an incident this should be uppermost in the mind of an investigator. I was called to a fire in the early hours in a south London boarding house where the fire brigade had discovered a dead and badly-burned body. When I arrived the fire had been extinguished and one of the fire brigade's own Fire Investigation Officers was present. We often worked closely and with mutual respect with these specialists. He and the uniform duty officer filled me in with the details as they knew them and he voiced the opinion that it looked accidental. The source of the fire seemed to be a dodgy gas oven where a pot had burned out, perhaps having been left unattended by the occupant, which went on to ignite soft furnishings in the small and squalid single room. The occupier was known by local officers to be a heavy drinker.

I had a quick look around and asked the photographer to take standard photos for the file. The deceased had been wrapped in a body bag while the fire-fighters doused the fire. I opened up the bag and saw, as expected, that the victim had suffered extreme burns throughout his upper body. He lay in a foetal position with both arms, and particularly his hands, in what is described in these circumstances as 'a pugilistic stance', in layman's terms adopting the stance of a boxer with arms up in a defensive, blocking stance with fists turned inwards. With the aid of a powerful torch (there was only emergency lighting in the house which was not very illuminating), I scanned the body looking for anything unusual or something that would assist with positive identification when I noticed one of his hands was wrapped around the handle of a large kitchen knife, partially burned, the blade of which was embedded up to the hilt in his sternum. As the scene was no longer accidental in my opinion and after updating the fire-fighter and duty officer I called out the MPFSL's FIU, a pathologist and SOCO, then informed the area on-call SIO that he had a 'sticker' (a suspicious death requiring full investigation). Post-mortem examination established the cause of death as stab wounds to the chest and MIT detectives went on to arrest and convict his murderer. You can never be too careful, particularly at arson scenes.

One of the closest venues to my then home address that I was called to was a public house in Chislehurst, Kent. It no longer exists and has been replaced by a pharmacy. I lived in nearby Orpington so on receipt of the out-of-hours call was on the scene quite quickly, so much so that the alleged female perpetrator was still on the premises awaiting transportation. The victim had been removed by paramedics but was found to be dead on arrival at the hospital nearby. It seemed that she was engaged as a barmaid at the pub and was in a relationship with the deceased who was the publican. According to her they'd spent the previous weekend enjoying each other sexually. Some years earlier the publican had been savagely beaten during a burglary at the premises which led him to illegally obtaining a handgun lest it should happen again. This he kept under a pillow on his bed.

The morning after this joint debauchery, probably fuelled by a rather heavy alcohol intake, the deceased had allegedly (according to the barmaid) told her she was a slut and was to pack her things up and get out of his pub immediately. An argument ensued that ended in two shots being fired from this revolver, one of which ended in the chest of the publican, causing his death. During a later interview she changed this version to one in which they were using the revolver as a sex toy and it just went off.

A PC who initially attended this incident had seized the weapon from the bed where it lay next to the barmaid so I secured it after making it safe, then started a detailed forensic examination of the bedroom but I couldn't find the alleged second spent bullet which had missed the deceased, although I located a ricochet mark on the ceiling. Not wishing to leave any stone unturned, I summoned a colleague from the MPFSL Firearms Team. After I briefed him he looked over the scene and drew my attention to the bottom drawer of a sideboard positioned opposite the bed which was slightly open by about half an inch. When we looked inside, there, sitting on top of some bedding, was my errant bullet head. He was able to provide expert evidence of the exact location where this bullet had been fired. It certainly wasn't where the perpetrator and the deceased had been entangled in bed as she was claiming, but from a point in the middle of the room. Bang goes the accidental discharge defence, if you'll pardon the expression.

Not far away and a few days later a fight ensued in an Orpington public house in which a member of the travelling community had an argument with a local and after a few punches were exchanged the traveller took a beating and left. At closing time the local involved in the fight left the premises and as he started to walk home a white van was driven from the pub car park and ran him down. Not satisfied with that, the driver reversed the vehicle over the prone body and then ran over him again as he made his way off. Again I was on scene quite quickly and with the pre-requested aid of a road accident collision expert from Traffic Branch examined the impact area and photographed tyre marks plus samples of debris for comparison with the suspect vehicle if/when it was traced.

A bizarre twist to this incident was that the victim was so badly injured he could not be taken to the local hospital as it didn't have the intensive medical facilities required, so he was airlifted by helicopter to find another suitable A&E premises. Would you believe it, as the crew flew this poor man over London, paramedics constantly contacting their HQ via radio, no A&E department was able to admit him. His journey ended (literally) at Leeds General Hospital where he succumbed to his injuries. The Leeds coroner was so incensed that no NHS vacancy could be found to treat the victim's life-threatening injuries that he refused to release the body to his south London equivalent. This meant that the SIO with me and the first PC on the scene who had assisted with the victim's emplacement on the helicopter had to travel to Leeds for the post mortem, the PC to formally identify the body to the pathologist as required by law. We all found it difficult to believe that nowhere else was available during the flight. Letters from the Leeds coroner to the London Ambulance Service and NHS requested answers to this unfortunate situation and senior personnel of both services were requested to attend the inquest and explain why. For the relatives of this tragedy this must have been a truly awful time. Could he have been saved if a nearer venue had been available? We'll never know for sure I'm afraid, but I believe this was a travesty of justice.

Not all crime scenes are what they appear to be at first sight so although every scene should be investigated to the nth degree, some need more of an 'out of the box' approach backed up by the investigator's experience. By way of example, one afternoon I was informed by phone of a suspicious death in a suburb of Croydon, south London, where a social worker had discovered an elderly female apparently dead in her home. Local uniform officers had attended and considered the circumstances were suspicious so the local CID had been alerted. I was engaged in an important case conference concerning a murder scene I'd dealt with recently that required my continued attendance so I requested that they contain the scene until I was able to attend. In the meantime I advised that they call in a local GP to formally establish death.

When I arrived I was aware of a large uniform presence in the vicinity engaged in house-to-house enquiries accompanied by the local CID. A Det Supt had been alerted after the GP confirmed the lady was dead but had concerns because of the presence of a head injury. This SIO was on scene and after a short conversation I learned that he was treating the incident as a possible burglary and assault due to the disarray in the room where the body was discovered, coupled with the lady's head wound. The Territorial Support Group (TSG), which is a mobile group of uniform officers drafted in from area resources to combat specific crime in particular areas, were operating nearby so the SIO rightly utilized them to speak to neighbours or passers-by to ascertain if anyone had seen or heard anything suspicious relative to the relevant address.

I noted how cold it was in the house and saw the deceased was lying in a foetal position on a bare floor beneath a table where several chairs had been overturned and placed around her. She looked frail and emaciated. Items of clothing lay beside her. She was minimally dressed in undergarments and I saw scratch marks on her legs and arms. Several cabinet drawers and doors of a Welsh dresser were open – all of these at a low level – and their contents strewn around the floor. Lying next to the deceased were several photographs from a photograph album. Her head wound was quite minimal but had bled and there was slight blood spattering on one of the open drawers.

I'd witnessed this kind of scenario before so I informed the SIO that I did not think this was a crime scene. To say the least, he was not convinced. How do you explain her head injury, her disturbed clothing, and the disruption to the furniture were among the queries he put to me. The on-call photographer arrived with a SOCO so I quickly briefed them, requesting the SOCO to prioritize examining all points of entry for evidence of forced entry and the photographer, with whom I'd covered many crime scenes before, to record the dining room and deceased in detail. That done, I went with the SIO to the kitchen and had a look in the fridge which was virtually empty apart from some mouldy butter and sour-smelling milk. A few cans of vegetables were the only foodstuffs in the cupboards. A sink contained several unwashed dishes with only a small amount of mouldy uneaten food adhering to them. A half-full cup of cold tea stood by a kettle. I was of the opinion that this was a classic case of hypothermia so I advised the SIO to restrict the house-to-house enquiries and contain it to when the lady had last been seen and her state of health at the time. I have to be honest, I had my fingers firmly crossed when I called this a non-suspicious death and while awaiting the arrival of the on-call pathologist who would have more in-depth experience of such occurrences (hopefully), I went over my reasoning in my head several times as well as with the SIO in answer to his numerous questions.

The SOCO did not find any evidence of forced entry which bolstered me somewhat. Hypothermia is quite common among the elderly when they cannot maintain their body heat or forget to do so when the weather is particularly cold. Add poor health and bad diet to this, and a form of dementia sets in. Research regarding survivors had revealed that such persons, although becoming dangerously cold, think they are hot so remove their clothing. I'd noted that this unfortunate lady had long fingernails that could have caused the scratches on her limbs as she undressed herself. She had formed a kind of nest with the furniture to hide in; again common with this ailment. In my opinion she'd opened the drawers and cupboards during more lucid spells in order to recall her identity or just to look at old photos. I was also aware that distinct ulcers would be present in the stomach lining in such cases.

As you can imagine, I was relieved in a professionally subdued way when the pathologist attended and after his own inspection agreed with my interpretation. It still all depended on the post-mortem findings, however. Sure enough, later that day the cause of death was confirmed as hypothermia. The SIO was impressed (his own words) because this saved him the not-so-little cost of a murder enquiry plus another drain on his limited staff resources. It didn't do my professional reputation any harm either. There's no substitute for experience.

Chapter 20

Beaten, Raped and Left to Die in Brixton

At around 7.00 am one day in February 1992 Ms Merlyn Nuttall, a young fashion designer, was standing at a bus stop in Effra Road, Brixton waiting for a bus to take her to work, like all the other commuters in the queue, when she became aware of a man in a tracksuit alongside her asking if she could help him. His pregnant girlfriend, he said, had fallen and he wanted Merlyn to stay with her while he called an ambulance. It was daylight, the street was busy with pedestrians, and traffic, as usual at this time of day, was heavy. He grabbed her arm, showed her a knife blade concealed in his other hand and led her to a nearby dilapidated three-storey building 4 or 5 yards across the pavement. She was so transfixed with fear and disbelief that she didn't cry out but went with him, aware that the knife blade was now stuck into her side. None of the others in the queue responded in any way. The man pushed her up to the top floor into an attic where you will not be surprised to learn there was no pregnant girlfriend.

Ms Nuttall then suffered a most horrific and brutal sexual attack. She was beaten, raped and forced to conduct sexual acts, then her attacker produced a length of cheese wire which he placed around her neck from behind and attempted to cut her throat. Trying to protect herself, she managed to insert the thumb of her right hand between the wire and her throat. The thumb was nearly severed, cut through to the bone. As she tried to fight him off and struggled to survive, he picked up a broken bottle and hacked away at her throat from behind. Understandably she lost consciousness.

She awoke with a start, not knowing how long she'd been unconscious, to the smell of burning and crackling of fire and soon became aware that he'd placed her clothing in a pile on top of her body and set it on fire. As she panicked and struggled he again jabbed at her neck, throat and head with the bottle. She decided that the only way she would survive was to feign death so she ignored the agonizing pain and stopped reacting to his beatings and bottle thrusts and went limp. After what must have seemed an age, she was aware that the room was filling with smoke so she got up, eventually opened the door and, devoid of any clothing, fell and slid down the stairs. She was now screaming for help, aware that her neck and throat were bleeding profusely, as was her right hand, and still terrified because she wasn't sure if her attacker had gone or not. Fire-fighters alerted to the fire found her in this tragic and dishevelled state. The rapid response of one of them who administered first aid and stemmed the blood flow from her neck and throat injuries undoubtedly saved her life. Her windpipe and bone were visible. Police officers who'd followed the fire engine to see if they could assist continued this sterling work and summoned an ambulance post-haste. The stalwart work of the hospital medical team also merits a mention.

When I got to the scene and was briefed by a local uniform sergeant who had set up a proper cordon it was obvious that this was going to be a lengthy forensic examination. I called in a photographer, fingerprint officer, a couple of SOCOs and some emergency lighting equipment, then informed the on-call SIO that I'd need an exhibit officer pronto because a full forensic examination of a three-storey building that was obviously a squat frequented by drug-users and had been subjected in part to a deliberately set fire was going to take more than a little time.

I recall a similar murder scene in a drug squat some months before in the wee small hours when I'd received a return phone call from a supervisor of the unit that we got in touch with to have lighting, forensic tents and similar equipment delivered. I'd rung his office requesting emergency lighting. Once I told him I was dealing with a murder, which was normally sufficient for the item to be packed into a van and delivered forthwith, he asked 'Why do you need lighting?' Initially perplexed and probably more than a little tired, I said something like 'Do you have any windows where you are, cause it's f***ing dark here' and immediately regretted it. Before he could respond I apologized and went on to say: 'There's no electric power available on the premises and there's a lot of syringes and sharps around so I want to make sure nobody gets one stuck in them while we examine around the corpse.' He responded 'Sorry mate, I just woke up and I'm new to this. I'll get it to you within the hour', and he did.

Here I was with yet another sad, macabre and tragic attempted murder. I'd just gone through a particularly busy and harrowing tour of on-call duties and the build-up of technically more demanding jobs, all of which required focused attention, and such dedication to detail had taken more of a toll on me than I was aware. It was of course the same for all my fellow LLOs. We all experienced busier than normal patches and it was during these that the camaraderie kicked in, and colleagues, who were themselves more than busy, would volunteer to help when and where possible.

As we worked Ms Nuttall's squalid and disgusting crime scene, taking special precautions because of the presence of sharps and other drugs paraphernalia, I sought the assistance of the FIU and a biologist from MPFSL to respectively bring their expertise regarding the fire source and blood distribution caused by the victim's blood being cast off onto the floor, walls and doors as the attacker repeatedly stabbed and jabbed her. The following day I also harnessed the volunteered services of my colleague Cliff as we split the house into sections to ensure that we missed nothing. Overall we took in excess of 150 exhibits that would be prioritized by me and the SIO as to which we felt would yield the most evidence in the shortest period of time in order to identify and apprehend the culprit. During this examination Cliff sawed off part of the stair banister that had given a positive reaction to a standard blood test indicating the presence of human blood and which the fingerprint officer thought may also provide relevant fingerprints. This item of evidence was subsequently the subject of a claim for compensation for damage made by the owners of the property who stated that as it was a listed building, their permission should have been sought prior to removal; another matter for the already busy SIO to deal with, which he could well have done without.

This is a classic example of Locard's Exchange Principle, well known and executed at virtually every crime scene by every forensic investigator worldwide. Frenchman Dr Edmond Locard (1877–1966) was a leading criminologist and pioneer in forensic science, dubbed 'the Sherlock Holmes of France', who in 1910 persuaded Lyon Police Force to establish the very first police laboratory with him as the lead scientist and from where he formulated the principle that 'every contact leaves a trace' which bears his name to this day. Rumour has it that the author Sir Arthur Conan Doyle, who created the fictional character of Sherlock Holmes, befriended Locard no doubt in order to pick his forensic brain for use in Sir Arthur's popular crime novels.

Examining large numbers of forensic exhibits takes up a lot of lab time and is expensive. As time goes on with no result, other forensic analytical methods, mostly very time-consuming, are adopted if the incident demands. Items were sent to other less busy laboratories but still nothing positive was gleaned. Eventually, using a new DNA identification process, biologists at MPFSL identified Ms Nuttall's blood and a latent fingerprint on a tissue/serviette which we recovered on the third and last day of our forensic examination. It was lying near the bottom of the stairwell where it had either fallen from the top floor or had been carried down and discarded by the attacker or Ms Nuttall herself. Specialist chemical treatment proved the print to be that of Anthony Ferrira. This put him within the premises at the same time as Ms Nuttall so he needed to be traced and brought in for questioning as a priority. If he had committed this awful deed, he needed to be removed from the streets of London where he was undeniably a serious threat to the public, especially females.

Ferrira (nicknamed 'Ripper') was a crack addict, pimp and total waste of space who had a dire criminal record including the sexual assault of a 13-year-old female and the manslaughter of a fellow prison inmate who he stabbed to death with scissors during a fight. When Ferrira was arrested and interviewed he denied all three charges of attempted murder, indecent assault and kidnapping of Ms Nuttall. It took the trial jury about two hours to find him guilty. He was sentenced to twenty years, eight years and five years respectively, to run concurrently, which meant a minimum of twenty years' imprisonment. An ideal candidate for euthanasia, in my opinion. All in all an excellent result brought about by a very professional crime scene examination, followed by first-class scientific analysis and grade 'A' detective work conducted by an MIT.

Should the reader be further interested in this atrocious crime, I recommend Merlyn Nuttall's autobiographic book outlining the brutality of the attack upon her and her amazing recovery, as well as her offer of advice on how to survive such trauma. Her courage and resilience is there for all to see in this remarkably frank work entitled *It Could Have Been You* published in 1998 by Virago Press.

Chapter 21

Teapot 1

An unwritten and generally unknown perk accorded the LLO is the authority to call out Teapot 1. The Met had its own catering service in those days, aptly named the Metropolitan Police Catering Service (MPCS), which provided a mobile canteen facility that could be summoned to any event or crime scene where Met staff had been detained or would be detained over a lengthy period of time and in sufficient numbers to warrant the expense and where it was not possible to obtain much-needed refreshments, especially during the night. The radio call sign for this sadly now defunct facility was 'Teapot 1'. I called them out on several occasions and once you got to know the lovely Irish lady who frequently answered the phone, you were asked if there was anything specific that you wished them to provide. Their menu ranged from tea, coffee, soup, soft drinks, water, fruit, sandwiches, biscuits and buns to hot cooked meals, all served with a cheery smile from their van parked just outside the police cordon.

I particularly recall ordering Teapot 1 to a fatal shooting of two men, a falling-out between rival major criminals apparently, in a south London street where myself, SOCO, photographer pals and the pathologist were working under a forensic tent for some time. I left the tent to collect more kit from my car only to find that nearly all the uniform cops who were supposed to be protecting the cordon and ensuring the public stayed away were crowded around the Teapot 1 mobile catering van that had arrived some ten minutes earlier. No-one had thought to let us know in the tent, even though I had summoned the refreshments myself. Thanks very much lads. To add insult to injury, as I approached the serving hatch to collect some hot drinks for my forensic mates I overheard a PC criticizing the hot pies that I had specifically asked Teapot 1 to bring. These were Scottish-style mutton pies that took me back to my youth in Fife and I'd recently enjoyed them at another major crime scene when MPCS had them on the menu. There's no accounting for taste, it seems.

My most memorable recollection of this fine service, however, was on a wet and dismal weekend when I was helping out a fellow Lab Sgt and long-term friend known to most simply by his initials 'PP'. He'd been the office manager in the MIT incident room dealing with the high-profile murder of Rachel Nickell before joining the LLO team. In the capacity of Lab Sgt he was dealing with a murder near Croydon where a female had been dismembered and body parts deposited in shallow graves around a local golf course. I was with a team extracting a couple of her limbs that were covered in plastic bags while PP dealt with the torso and other pieces discovered in another part of the course. The crime scene was split in this way to avoid issues of cross-contamination. As we toiled, photog tapped me on the shoulder and pointed towards a hill behind us where two electric golf carts were slowly descending. One was driven by PP with a passenger unknown to us clutching a number of small white cardboard boxes. The other was driven by a DC from an MIT which, as it drew closer, revealed the lovely Irish lady from Teapot 1 sitting in the front passenger seat with a tea urn nestled in her lap. Another of her colleagues in the back seat held a selection of snacks. A truly amusingly unusual and most welcome sight that none of those present are likely ever to forget. Well done PP, and of course well done the fine staff of MPCS and Teapot 1.

Chapter 22

Crime Scene Examination on Wimbledon Common

Some five months later, still trying like all my LLO colleagues to keep apace of the murders and major enquiries that were coming our way all too regularly I received a call, the eventual circumstances of which stay with me to this day and caused me a lot of soul-searching, concern and discussions with fellow professionals for a long time afterwards when trying to determine if anything had been missed in the initial extensive crime scene examination and related enquiries.

It was about 10.30 am on a warm, bright and sunny July day in 1992 when an architect taking his daily constitutional on Wimbledon Common came across the inert and heavily bloodstained body of Rachel Nickell. The hue and cry went up and as I was the on-call Lab Sgt for that area it very quickly came to me. I was already heading to a location not far off to check on the progress of another murder investigation so I simply changed direction and headed for the rendezvous point (RVP) in a public car park near the popular Windmill Café. My mind was abuzz with options as I tried to prioritize how I would engage with an incident in such a large communally-used area and consider what assistance and logistics I'd need to call in and in what order.

When I arrived at the RVP I was briefed by a uniform skipper (sergeant) who'd cordoned off the immediate area near to where I would find Rachel's body and had done a damn good job in enlisting park rangers and all available uniform staff from nearby police stations to contain this larger than normal crime scene. Not an easy task for an area of some 11,040 acres (460 hectares) where it was subsequently estimated that upwards of 500 people had been dog-walking, jogging, horse-riding or otherwise innocently enjoying the space. During this briefing I noticed a very young boy being held by a female uniform PC near to an ambulance and was told he was thought to be the son of the victim. I could see he had small scratches on his face and was obviously quite distressed as he cuddled into the officer. I had a quick chat with

131

her as she entered the ambulance to take him to the local hospital for a medical check-up and reminded her to ensure that his clothing was secured and discreet hair combings and swabs taken from him for consideration of later forensic examination. Another PC was looking after what was believed to be their pet dog.

With the skipper I retraced the path he'd taken earlier and walked carefully to where the lady's body was lying just off the path beneath small birch trees. I immediately saw that this was going to be a difficult crime scene to organize and examine. Her pale body could be seen from some distance away, which was alarming. I called in the duty pathologist, photographer and all available SOCOs as I took stock of the situation, using the waiting time to scour the immediate area around her body to see if any fibres, hairs or anything alien to the shrubbery was evident. There were signs of a struggle. Foot imprints, hoof marks, paw marks and different types of tyre marks were in abundance. Rachel lay on her left side in a sort of foetal position with her arms and hands pulled up towards her neck and face. Her jeans and panties had been pulled down over her shoes, which probably prevented them being removed altogether, and her heavily bloodstained T-shirt was dishevelled, exposing her midriff region. There were multiple deep stab wounds in her neck and upper chest area. All of this raised the following questions:

- How could this happen in broad daylight in an area frequented by so many people?
- What sort of a creature could do this in the presence of her child and a dog?
- How would this affect the little boy?
- What terror had Rachel gone through in trying to protect her child, never mind protecting herself?

No sane person could have done this. We had to stop this monster, and sooner rather than later. To say the least, the perpetrator was an extreme danger to the public, especially women, while still at large.

In order to have a complete examination kit and sufficient consumable items in my murder bag for when the pathologist and the rest of the team arrived, I returned to my car and started to pick out what I needed. A couple of DSs from the neighbouring area ('V' Division) that I knew and had noticed earlier popped over to my car. They were waiting to see if they could be of any help to the MIT when they arrived. After exchanging a few pleasantries I headed back to the body and remember one of them saying: 'Rather you than me, Ron.' How right they were. It was plain to see by this time that some members of the press were arriving. Apart from local newspaper reporters, large TV and radio vans were vying for positions in the car park, their crews setting up recording and camera equipment with reporters already chatting to people in and around the café; a point to bear in mind as we moved around the crime scene.

Dr Richard 'Dick' Shepherd, a hugely experienced Home Office criminal pathologist with whom I'd worked on many cases before, arrived and confirmed life extinct as we began examining Ms Nickell's body. As the force photographer went about his quotidian business, a couple of SOCOs began the thankless but necessary task of obtaining plaster-cast impressions of any suspect marks in the immediate proximity and the possible path taken by Rachel and her attacker. A child's T-shirt, later identified as belonging to her 2-year-old son Alex, was found a short distance away on the main path. It was most probably here that the attack began. While Dick examined and counted approximately forty-nine stab wounds, any one of which in the neck area could have proved fatal, I took hair combings, outer clothing tapings, blood swabs and sexual swabs from various parts of Rachel's body. Upon completion of this grim but essential task, we placed her in a body bag and carefully carried her out to a private ambulance for transportation to the local mortuary, where later that day Dick would carry out a detailed post mortem and he and I would extract any further swabs deemed necessary. A designated CID exhibit officer from the MIT would record, collect and package all exhibits for us to prioritize after discussion on a Lab form before submission to MPFSL for forensic analysis.

Incidentally, the reader might be interested to know that Dr Shepherd has written an excellent autobiography entitled *Unnatural Causes: The Life and Many Deaths of Britain's Top Forensic Pathologist* published in 2018 by Penguin in which he admits to having to deal with many demons that caused him personal dismay and concern throughout his lengthy career, during which he dealt with an unbelievable 23,000 post mortems worldwide. Professor Sue Black, a highly-experienced forensic anthropologist and herself an autobiographical author of *All That Remains* refers to Dick's book as 'Heart-wrenchingly honest'. Although I had the privilege to work alongside Dick in a great many post mortems, crime scenes and murders abroad, I was never aware of his internal conflicts. No doubt this was indeed the case for other professionals who regularly engaged with him. I found the book revealing and the frank way in which Dick explains his lifelong search for truth is both fascinating and compelling.

On completion of the biological analysis of all exhibits submitted thus far, only DNA relevant to Ms Nickell was identified. There was no alien DNA in any of the samples we'd taken. I discussed in depth with the forensic biologists who conducted the examination to see if we could do anything more. MPFSL employed some of the finest forensic scientists in the country and possessed the most up-to-date scientific equipment. They tried a new and relatively untested DNA identification system, but again it took us nowhere.

Back in the incident room, the MIT staff were struggling to keep up with the flow of information coming in from the great British public. It was normal to find fifteen to twenty staff setting up a new incident room, but on this occasion something like thirty to forty officers and admin staff were drafted in. Computers and ancillary IT equipment were already being delivered in order to install the relatively new Home Office Large Major Enquiry System (HOLMES) which is a boon to a large and complicated investigation. However, it takes a little time to get going so any information obtained in the first day or so of any major investigation has to be handwritten, the original filed and a copy handed to the detectives tasked with chasing it up and interviewing the source. This is known as an 'action'. Officers can be issued several actions at a time and they all have to be written up and put back into the system either completed or for further action as soon as possible. This takes time and depends on staff resources available to the SIO. This particular investigation and following re-investigation would result in the taking of 2,893 statements, 1,676 interviews were recorded and an overall total of 6,761 potential witnesses were seen. Thirty-three arrests would be made. An extremely busy period indeed for all involved.

In excess of 700 'actions' were created in the first two weeks of this inquiry. Among these would be well-meaning members of the public who may not have anything to take the inquiry further but wished to help in any way they could, as well as the annoying and frustrating hoax callers who unfortunately are always drawn to high-profile crime investigations and who we can well do without. All would have to be traced and seen. In the past, mediums and psychics have contacted incident rooms to pass on their 'sightings'. Silly though this may seem, they also have to be eliminated. Separating the wheat from the chaff early in these circumstances is an art. Photofit (facial composite) likenesses created by witnesses were circulated. Officers trawled local and national police records to try to identify any known suspects. Informants were visited. TV, radio, newspapers and any media outlet that could assist was contacted by Scotland Yard's media communication liaison team at the Press Bureau.

Soon a suspect was evolving from a combination of local intelligence, Photofits and witness statements. His name was Colin Stagg. It would ultimately prove unfortunate for him that he also fitted a criminal profile of Rachel's attacker compiled by Paul Britton, the self-proclaimed foremost criminal psychologist in the UK who was lending his professional weight to the investigation. Criminal profiling is an acceptable aid and can be an invaluable investigative tool. It's been available for some time and to my personal knowledge used by SIOs in several major investigations. The profile is intended to corroborate other tangible evidence in the case and should, when done properly, assist investigators to look in the right direction for their quarry and not waste valuable time pursuing every Tom, Dick or Harry suspect. It should produce clues as to the habits and lifestyle of a suspect and lead towards identifying their status, thinking process and behaviour. Physical descriptions and clothing will have come from witness statements. In this case Britton would have been asked if Stagg fitted his profile of Ms Nickell's attacker. One can only assume he said yes.

I attended a number of meetings with the SIO and his management team in which we discussed the up-to-date position of various exhibits still undergoing scientific examination in MPFSL and other forensic labs with the intention of what to do next exhibit-wise. It was decided that Stagg would be arrested, brought in for questioning and his home searched. Because I'd covered the murder scene and post mortem and had discussed the type of weapon used with the pathologist, it was agreed that I should form part of the house-search team. This was carried out shortly afterwards. His home was unusually decorated with Satanic-style almost 'cave-like' drawings of animals and birds on matt blackboard walls in a rear room where a large occult cross was drawn on the floor. It gave the impression of an altar of some sort. After full video and still photography was completed, various items of clothing and utensils of a survivalist nature as well as a type of wooden knobkerrie club were seized for forensic comparison.

It's fair to say that as time went by and nothing of a positive nature came from the numerous forensic examinations undertaken by MPFSL and others I, like many officers involved, became more and more frustrated and disappointed. A second post mortem was undertaken, which is unusual, but again to no avail. I attended even more meetings with the MIT management as we went over all aspects of the investigation. I was asked repeatedly if anything further could be done. I even brought along one of the lead biologists from MPFSL to one of these meetings to explain in detail that what had been done was all that could be done at that time. It was one of the benefits of having a LLO office within the MPFSL where we could literally chat with scientists as they worked on exhibits from our cases. In this way we built up good professional relationships with one another. Mass DNA screening of all males living in and around Wimbledon Common was begun, especially those who had previous convictions or were suspected of crimes of a sexual nature, of which there were more than 100. These would be compared against all suspect DNA held on the national DNA database.

Meanwhile the case against Stagg continued to gather momentum and took another unusual tack. I had no involvement in the ensuing undercover (UC) aspect of the case, I'm glad to say, which ended with severe criticism and condemnation of both the manner in which police handled the covert operation and the criminal profiler's tactics when the case against Stagg collapsed. This greatly disappointed the SIO and his team, as it did me. His Lordship Mr Justice Ognall, sitting in the Central Criminal Court at the Old Bailey, was quoted as using the terms 'thoroughly reprehensible' and 'deceptive conduct of the grossest kind' with reference to the UC operation. A UC operation requires authority at the highest level at Scotland Yard as well as the agreement of senior figures in the CPS who make the ultimate decisions regarding procedures to be adopted and ultimately whether a case should go to court or not. Therefore these inimitable personages must have decreed the use of Britton and the UC operation as worthy.

I'm no expert in criminal profiling but I do have a basic understanding of the concept. In my personal opinion Paul Britton was allowed too much control of this covert operation which led the team down the path of suspecting Stagg as the only suspect instead of the best one available at that time. Britton's alleged compilation of scripts for the UC officer's conversations and the content of letters between her and Stagg were taking things too far in my estimation, coming too close to being *agent provocateur* which is rarely acceptable in British criminal courts. In layman's terms, this equates to 'a person employed to lead others, by pretending sympathy with them, into committing unlawful acts.' To be fair Britton denied this, but then he would, wouldn't he? Who else could or would have proffered this line of advice? I know that many officers involved in this inquiry felt as I did.

For a more detailed account of the UC operation which came under severe criticism, in fact condemnation, by the judge at Stagg's trial plus Paul Britton's involvement in the investigation I would direct the reader to former DI Keith Pedder's book titled *The Rachel Files: The Untold Secrets of the Rachel Nickell Investigation* published in 2002 by John Blake Publishing Ltd. Keith was in charge of the UC operation.

Stagg would go on to receive sizeable financial compensation from the Met, but his life was unsurprisingly in ruins. He received death threats, the Employment Agency couldn't find anyone willing to give him a job and his brief, tumultuous marriage ended in an acrimonious divorce. The UC officer didn't fare too well either. She left the Met after a lengthy period of stress-related sick leave. Keith Pedder also left the Met prematurely after periods of stress-related illness. In his next career as a private investigator his situation was not helped by being the subject of criminal investigation for corruption, although his trial collapsed within days. Paul Britton fell off the police radar and was not involved with any Met major crime investigations thereafter to my knowledge.

For the record, over the next few years the Met undertook a series of extensive and expensive reviews which were conducted by several different SIOs and teams who were in no way involved in the original enquiries of several murders that were still unsolved, the murder of Rachel Nickell being one of them, but it wasn't until 2004 that an independent laboratory (Forensic Alliance) which had formulated a new DNA identification process positively identified microscopic particles from a swab taken from items belonging to convicted murderer Robert Napper within hair combings from Rachel's son Alex. The advances of science had caught up with him at last, thanks mainly to the determination of dedicated forensic scientists but also because of the hard work and perseverance of many Met CID officers. It took another year for this identification to be confirmed. This is another fine example of Locard's Exchange Principle (see Chapter 20).

By this time I'd resigned from the Met after completing almost thirty-five years' service and was engaged in war crime investigations with the UN International Criminal Tribunal for the former Yugoslavia (ICTY) in The Hague, Netherlands. A pal still serving as a CID officer in the Met contacted me there and passed on the good news. It was very good news indeed, especially so when I learned that the evidential link to Napper being Rachel's attacker came from Alex's hair combings which I'd directed should be taken. I shared a pint or two with him when I next returned home on leave. Rachel's murder and the extensive crime scene work it occasioned definitely lost me more sleep over the years than any other case in which I was involved by a long chalk. I recently (in 2018) appeared on a TV documentary presented by Fiona Bruce as she sought to ascertain the points learned by the Met and the impact Rachel's murder had on those directly involved over the past twenty-five years, especially those police officers involved. During the filming of this programme and discussions with the presenter, a great many of the conflicting emotions I experienced during and after my dealings with the murder came back to haunt me once more.

Napper was already serving a life sentence in a secure mental establishment for the rape and murder of young mother Samantha Bisset and the sexual assault and murder of her 4-year-old daughter Jazmine in their home in Plumstead, south London, in November 1993 due to his fingerprints being found within the premises. To my knowledge, he had not been a major suspect in the Nickell murder. When Napper eventually came to trial for Rachel's murder in 2008 he was deemed *non compos mentis* (of unsound mind); quite simply unable to stand trial due to his mental state. A plea of guilty to the lesser charge of manslaughter was submitted as a result of admissions on his behalf by his QC and agreed by the court. The learned judge ordered that he be remanded indefinitely in Broadmoor Hospital, the UK's most secure mental institution, where hopefully he will remain for the rest of his miserable existence.

Chapter 23

Who Dares Wins

One evening a doctor on duty in the A&E unit of a Croydon hospital called police because of misgivings he had regarding a dead infant who'd just been brought in by the young parents. I held a short conversation with the night-duty CID officer, as a result of which we organized a post-mortem examination for the following morning at the local mortuary. A CID officer from the MIT who had obtained some knowledge of the case and a police photographer joined the pathologist and me for this function. The pathologist was of the opinion that the baby had been severely beaten about the face and body. Noticing small bruises on the ankle areas also led him to believe that the child had been held by the ankles and swung forcibly against a hard surface, thus causing fatal damage to the cranium. We had another murder. The parents had been held overnight at Croydon police station as they'd given different versions of how their child had received these fatal injuries.

I met up with the designated SIO and we agreed that a full forensic examination of the parents' address should be a priority. Taking along an exhibit officer and the photographer, I made arrangements for a local SOCO to meet us at the premises. This very small flat was extremely warm, the heat coming from an electric bar fire left switched on in the lounge. We had begun a systematic examination when my attention was drawn to an overall smell of damp, and recent paintwork was evident on a lounge wall against which stood a child's cot. Above the cot was a large poster of an SAS trooper in full combat gear that looked out of place. We took it down and saw that the wall behind was tacky to the touch. White paint stuck to the finger. We took swabs and carefully cleaned away the recent paintwork which revealed a circular indentation. Repeatedly photographing and swabbing this area, we slowly uncovered a screwed-up ball of papier-mâché consistency. We painstakingly removed this intact and the SOCO made a synthetic cast of the slightly larger than fist-sized indentation. When set, we took the cast to the mortuary where we met up with the pathologist who placed it over the dead baby's head. It was a perfect fit. We took Polaroid pictures of this procedure so that we could share it with the SIO immediately. Further questioning of the parents established that the infant had been beaten and indeed swung against the wall above the cot as described by the pathologist. The couple had panicked and carried out the repairs we'd found, leaving their dead child in a buggy by the fire not only to keep the body warm but also to dry the paintwork. Their only discrepancy was that they each accused the other of the assault.

They maintained this stance at their trial. The CPS chose not to charge them with murder, so much lesser criminal charges were preferred which ultimately led to both being convicted. Both parents had learning difficulties and were really rather pathetic individuals; this is probably why they only received suspended prison sentences. Although a tragic and sad investigation, it was satisfying to have been part of a team that provided evidence of how this unfortunate infant had met a brutal death. In other words we had given the murdered child a voice and that was most satisfying. In fact this was really our main aim as we investigated every homicide, regardless of whether it was of a domestic nature or on a much larger scale in war crime investigations, of which more is to follow.

Chapter 24

Political Assassination in Sri Lanka

Only a few days after dealing with the crime scene at the notorious fatal stabbing of Stephen Lawrence in Well Hall Road, New Eltham in south London in April 1993 and effectively removing myself from continuing my involvement with that enquiry, I received a call that led me to Sri Lanka with an SIO and supporting DI nicknamed 'Ships' plus Dr Dick Shepherd, the ever-helpful and diligent pathologist with whom I'd worked at the Rachel Nickell murder scene and many others. This was due to a request from the Sri Lankan government who needed an independent investigation into the recent fatal shooting of a politician. The SIO – a proud Welshman named Alec Edwards – had been my DS during my first tour on the Flying Squad.

We got together as arranged in the Air Lanka lounge at Heathrow Airport where a member of the FCO (Foreign and Commonwealth Office) briefed us on the political and security situation in Sri Lanka given the ongoing war with Tamil terrorists. As the SIO, Alec had been briefed in more detail as to the incident we were to investigate. After some excellent hospitality from our hosts we took up our comfortable business-class seats for the trip to Colombo, the capital of Sri Lanka, all paid for by the Sri Lankan authorities. We had expected a low-key reception on arrival, as is the habit with such Scotland Yard foreign trips, but walking off the plane we were confronted by a national TV crew in the company of senior Sri Lankan police officers. Alec wasn't impressed. He wasn't alone. We were driven to a large secure hotel in Colombo where we were briefed in more detail and met our personal protection team (PROT) who would be with us 24/7. We each had two armed minders drawn from the ranks of the police, army and Air Force, plus three drivers. It became obvious as we were driven around that these were not discreet or covert vehicles. From the looks on pedestrians' faces and the way other drivers in Colombo gave us a wide berth, they obviously knew that these were government vehicles. If they knew, so would the Tamil terrorists.

Politician Lalith Athulathmudali had been shot at close range while giving a speech during a public political rally two days before in the outskirts of the capital by a man who nonchalantly emerged from the audience smoking a cigarette, then jumped up onto the podium and carried out the deed. The assailant was chased by police and security personnel who fired shots at him. He ran around a building where those pursuing him inexplicably stopped their pursuit. His dead body was discovered much later by municipal workers in a seated position leaning against a wall at the side of the building towards which he'd last been seen running. He apparently bore four bullet wounds to his back and held an automatic pistol in his lap. Police claimed he possessed ID in the name of Suppiah with an address in the Jaffna region. A cyanide capsule had also allegedly been found on his body. The local pathologist reported that apart from the gunshot wounds, he may have died of cyanide poisoning. We had been informed in an earlier briefing that it was the practice of Tamil terrorists to carry cyanide capsules when on certain missions. The men wore them inserted in the slots of their shirt collars where stiffeners are normally inserted, and the females wore them as a necklace charm.

Accompanied by a Sri Lankan police DCI who headed up their Forensic Unit, we viewed the crime scene. I recall that it was extremely humid and as I opened up my murder kit the heavens opened. I have a treasured photo of this DCI walking alongside me at the crime scene holding an umbrella over us (see photo plate section). I took some Polaroid shots, then swabs of blood smears on the wall where the assailant had been found. Upon completion, we went to the Sri Lanka Police HQ to secure the exhibits. I'd brought state-of-the-art self-sealing, see-through evidence bags from MPFSL but because of the humidity they wouldn't seal. The sticky tape with which I was issued was also useless. I asked the local DCI what his chaps used, so we went to his office where he handed me a roll of brown wrapping paper, a ball of string, a stick of red sealing wax and some safety matches. You can imagine my reaction. However comical these old-fashioned items seemed, they did the trick. As expected, I received a bit of a ribbing from my scientist buddies when I subsequently returned to MPFSL.

Dick and I carried out a post mortem the following day, the local pathologist having shared her report with us. She had only partially completed her examination because she was informed that a Scotland Yard team had been summoned. As Dick commenced an external inspection of the cadaver, we both noticed small glass fragments in the mouth. At the same time we detected the slight but telltale scent of almonds indicating the presence of cyanide, so I took an oral swab. The problem was, however, that without a control sample of known cyanide I had nothing with which to compare it. Neither Dick nor I had any experience of cyanide poisoning other than what we'd read or been told during forensic presentations. Dick also removed a small-calibre projectile from the spinal column near the coccyx which inexplicably had rested just under the surface of the epidermis. Usually this would have penetrated further. We asked the senior Sri Lankan police officers present if they could explain, but it seemed they couldn't (or wouldn't) confirm whether it was a police officer or personal bodyguard of the murdered politician who had shot the alleged assassin, a tad unusual given the sensitivity of this incident. We had been informed that both parties had pursued and fired at the assassin as he fled. Hopefully a ballistic comparison of this projectile and the weapons known to have been fired would clarify the situation. The good Dr Shepherd offered to conduct a further detailed post mortem on the murdered politician, but this was declined with no reason given.

We later joined our other team members who had been conducting enquiries elsewhere to discuss our findings and update our hosts. I mentioned my doubts in determining cyanide poisoning due to the lack of a control sample, and a senior Sri Lankan police officer present told us he could help. He took me to his office where in a cabinet drawer he showed me a tray of glass phials containing clear liquid sitting on a bed of cotton wool with another layer of cotton wool on top. He told me these were cyanide capsules intercepted from a Tamil terrorist source and invited me to select one as a control. It was the first and only time I handed a sealed and very well-packaged exhibit to a British Airways pilot, against signature, in order that he deliver same to a police officer at Heathrow Airport, who by arrangement would ensure that it was submitted to MPFSL. The lab later confirmed that the swab did contain cyanide, as did the glass phial. One of the many advantages of the LLO being an experienced detective as well as a forensic investigator is that on foreign trips when the forensic phase is complete he reverts to a standard DS role and assists with interviews, statement-taking and other general investigative duties as I did here.

A member of staff of the British Embassy in Colombo contacted us and made Alec aware that the FCO were concerned for our personal safety. President Ranasinghe Premadasa was due to speak, and probably go walkabout, at a major political rally in the capital on 1 May as was his habit. In the past this date had been a spark to ignite serious civil disturbance, violence and bombings. We were advised to vacate Colombo for a few days just in case, which advice we readily took.

Our hosts placed us in a good standard hotel well out of the capital and rather fortunately near the sea in Yala National Park. It was closed to the public due to ongoing repairs and redecoration. We occupied several comfortable chalets in the grounds with our PROT nearby as always. We took advantage of our enforced break by enjoying swimming in the beautifully clear warm sea, a visit to an elephant sanctuary and a trip to a turtle sanctuary where we purchased buckets of day-old turtles and released them into the sea. Local fishermen used to dig the eggs up after their mothers had laid them in their thousands on the beach and sold them for food. This didn't help in preserving the species, so the sanctuary paid the fishermen above the going rate to bring them to the sanctuary.

This was an amazing experience as the little blighters often turned back towards land, even after we'd placed them in the shallows several times. Their biggest danger, believe it or not, was from adult turtles that ate a considerable number of them in their earliest days. Back in the sanctuary we saw a large female adult albino turtle that had been rescued as she wouldn't survive in the wild. Tourists made a donation to take a photo with her. Some actually picked her up by the shell and held her in front of themselves for the photo. That was quite a feat as she was a big heavy girl. One not-so-bright lady turned the turtle around to get a photo of her kissing it when it bit into her nose, causing her severe injury. These turtles use their beaks to prise crustaceans off coral reefs and crush them open, for goodness sake. You can imagine what damage it would do to a human nose. As a result there was a large poster cautioning tourists against kissing said turtle. I felt a bit sorry for this lovely creature all alone in a small tank but I suppose the alternative was much worse.

Our R&R was not to last too long. Our protectors received a radio message from their HQ on 1 May to the effect that President Premadasa had been assassinated and many others killed in a bomb blast. Arrangements were made to return us to Colombo and assist with that incident. We switched on the TV and witnessed the carnage and mayhem caused by the explosion. Unbelievably a senior Sri Lankan police officer lifted up a decapitated human head by the hair, showed it to the TV camera and asked (according to our PROT colleagues) if any viewer could identify the owner who was suspected of detonating a suicide vest and causing the fatal explosion.

Because the roads between Yala and Colombo would now be subject to heavily-armed roadblocks manned by police and military personnel suspecting a Tamil incursion, our protection team feared that a convoy of three white unmarked cars would be in danger of receiving fire from trigger-happy and nervous personnel manning them. It would also be dark soon when there was a tendency for them to shoot first and ask questions later. We'd delay until daylight. I managed to speak with the Sri Lankan police forensic team DCI and asked if he could ensure that the crime scene was secured so we could begin a full forensic examination on arrival. He confirmed that he would.

It took us a while to get to Colombo, having to travel slowly and treat each of many roadblocks with utmost caution, but we made it unscathed. To our disappointment and disbelief the bodies, parts of bodies and general debris from the bomb blast area had been literally shovelled into a truck and delivered to a mortuary where they were unceremoniously dumped in the yard. To say the least, this went against the grain and defied all logic. Sri Lankan police were well-trained and adhered to British protocols for forensic investigations which they inherited when Sri Lanka was a colonial protectorate known as Ceylon before independence in 1972.

I spent a very unpleasant time picking through this pile of body parts assisting Sri Lankan police colleagues and mortuary staff and with difficulty eventually managed to identify a limb from the president, mainly due to an inscribed watch on the wrist. DNA samples were taken from the head shown on TV the day before, as well as from many other cadavers. A senior Sri Lankan police officer I'd come to know quite well informed me that police had indeed requested that the crime scene be guarded and secured until our return from Yala, but this was countermanded by the national security agency who overruled the police and ordered the site cleared forthwith. This did not make sense.

We learned that President Premadasa had indeed gone walkabout during his political rally in Colombo when a youth rode a bicycle up to his car and dismounted. He walked towards the president, but was stopped by a security agent. A valet in the president's employ told the agent to let this youth through as he was a friend. They did so, and it seems that as he reached the president and opened his arms to embrace him, the youth detonated a suicide bomb he was wearing, killing the president, himself, the valet and sixteen other senior military, police and politicians in the entourage. We were also informed of the presence of a cyanide capsule in the mouth of the bomber.

Sri Lankan police identified the bomber as 23-year-old Kulaveerasingam Veerakumar nicknamed 'Babu' and a resident of Jaffna. The following day at the request of the Sri Lankan police I went with a combined military and police armed convoy to a house in Jaffna identified as Babu's home. As the military commander deployed his heavily-armed troops, I was told to be as quick as possible because Jaffna was a hotbed of Tamil terrorist activity. Word of our presence would soon get out and snipers or bombers may target us. The Sri Lankan police SOCO and I were very brief. I seized a hairbrush and comb from the bathroom of this basic single-roomed residence, while my colleague lifted finger marks and took a few swabs. Safely ensconced in our armoured vehicle, we returned to Colombo without incident, quietly relieved but sweating profusely under our heavy flak jackets and not just because of the heat and humidity.

Our hosts cordially invited us to attend the funeral of their late president, an invitation that we gratefully accepted. Along with many national and international dignitaries and VIPs, we shared a grandstand view of the magnificently ornate funeral pyre which had been meticulously constructed in which to cremate him. It was a truly unique occasion. We departed Sri Lanka, in my opinion not quite agreeing with the Sri Lankan government's interpretation of the facts as presented to us surrounding the murder of politician Athulathmudali, but from my perspective I'd learned a great deal as a result of this most interesting forensic experience. DNA extracted from exhibits recovered from Babu's address did in fact identify him as the bomber responsible for the assassination of President Premadasa and the murder of seventeen others, plus of course his own suicide.

Chapter 25

Provisional Irish Republican Army (PIRA) Bombs a Bus in Aldwych

I was about to go to bed for the night shortly after 11.00 pm one February evening in 1996 when my job phone rang. A bomb had just gone off on a London bus in a street in Aldwych near The Strand in central London which was my old stomping ground when I was stationed at Bow Street nick earlier in my career. At least one person was presumed dead and several others seriously injured. I was told that traffic in the area was severely congested so I might want to seek assistance when I drew near in order to reach the RVP. I was living in Kent at the time so it would take me about an hour to drive to the scene. The duty photographer and a SOCO had already been alerted by anti-terrorist officers who assumed responsibility for such incidents.

As I reached the north end of the Old Kent Road, traffic was backing up and almost at a complete standstill. I decided to drive over Tower Bridge where traffic may be lighter, then try to get near the scene via City of London streets. 'Road Closed' signs were placed at traffic lights, but as there was almost no other traffic I carefully drove through. All of a sudden I saw something rebound off my windscreen and heard a loud bang as I crossed a set of traffic lights. Looking around, I saw a City of London PC striding swiftly towards me looking less than friendly. I can't remember his exact words, but they were something like: 'Can't you read? The road's closed. What makes you think you can just drive through?' I flashed my warrant card and told him I was endeavouring to make my way to the bombed bus in Aldwych to take charge of the crime scene and I assumed the 'Road Closed' signs were in place because of this incident. It turned out that they were. As he retrieved his truncheon, which he'd thrown and had hit my windscreen 'to gain my attention', he summoned a City police traffic motorcyclist to escort me to the scene. I thanked him, we shook hands, then I followed the traffic cop on blues and twos right to the crime scene cordon.

The carnage was incredible. The front of the bus was virtually destroyed and extraordinarily part of the roof of the top deck rested in a tree. There was considerable damage to buildings and windows to the nearside of the vehicle, while remarkably trees appeared undamaged on the opposite side of the street. Most of my technical forensic specialists were on scene, setting up their kits like the true professionals they are. Similarly, uniform officers at the scene had been busy and put in a good cordon and also summoned emergency lighting and other equipment. A Force Medical Examiner (FME) had already attended and pronounced life extinct from one body lying near the bottom of the stairway. This I would later determine to be the bomber. I could see that both of his lower limbs were missing and other serious body injuries were evident. I was made aware that a couple of passengers and the driver of the bus had been taken to the nearby St Thomas' Hospital along with people in a car near to the bus when the bomb went off at 2238 hours GMT. Police had not received any warning, so although initially the Provisional Irish Republican Army (PIRA) was the main suspected terrorist organization responsible, an open-minded approach was required.

At some stage PCs at the cordon told us that hot drinks and grub were available. This was much needed and would give those of us involved in the forensic examination an opportunity to collectively appraise our progress as well as take refreshments, so we decided to have a short break and were logged out of the crime scene. Just south of the cordon in The Strand a Salvation Army mobile canteen van was parked at the kerbside with a bunch of uniform cops standing around the rear, steaming paper cups in hand. On our approach the lady serving beckoned us over, having noted our telltale white paper suits, and said: 'Come on lads, let forensics through. I'm sure they really need a cuppa.' She was spot on. I cannot praise the Salvation Army enough for this facility, which they voluntarily roll out to many serious incidents to provide sustenance and a bit of a much-needed and welcome break to all emergency services personnel at the worst of times. Well done them.

We painstakingly processed the scene and established that the bomb had exploded in a briefcase carried by the bomber as he descended from the top deck. I was much later informed that it was probable that he was going to place it in a litter bin at the entrance to the Law Courts in The Strand where, had it exploded at 1000 hours the following morning, untold death and destruction would have occurred. I heard my name called out during this phase of the detailed examination and saw standing outside the cordon near a PC tasked with keeping a record of comings and goings the legendary Commander John Grieve, MPhil, CBE, QPM, who was in charge of Scotland Yard's Anti-Terrorist Branch (SO13), known affectionately to all ranks simply as 'JG'. I'd known JG from my early days in the Flying Squad and he was my DI on 11 Squad during my second tour in that esteemed unit at Tower Bridge. He is the most respected and admired detective with whom I've ever had the privilege to work and I'm proud to count him as a friend. His work ethic, forward thinking, drive, leadership and mental capacity are second to none, as a search of his achievements listed in Wikipedia and elsewhere will confirm.

Suitably attired in a protective suit, overshoes and surgical gloves to prevent contamination, JG came on board and I briefed him as to our findings. Close inspection of the body had revealed that the bomber was carrying a Walther PPK automatic 9mm pistol. This was unusual. Hitherto PIRA bombers had normally worked in pairs, one being an armed 'minder'. Bizarrely the man's wristwatch was still working. Unlike in most whodunnit stories, it had not stopped at the time of the explosion. His lower limbs were recovered some distance from the blast; one had actually been blown into the side panel of another PSV (Public Service Vehicle) travelling along The Strand south of the bombed bus. Along with all other body parts, these were placed in a body bag and removed to the local mortuary where the following day I attended the post-mortem examination which was carried out by the late great Dr Iain West. Iain recorded that death would have been 'virtually instantaneous'. Apart from standard post-mortem samples, fingerprints were taken to assist with identification.

The Explosives Officer believed that the bomb consisted of 5lb of Semtex plastic explosive set off by a twenty-four-hour timing device. Either this device was faulty or the bomb was poorly assembled, causing it to detonate earlier than intended. The bomber was positively identified as Edward O'Brien. Anti-terrorist colleagues ultimately searched his London address and recovered 33lb of Semtex, twenty timing devices, four detonators and a quantity of 9mm ammunition that would fit the Walther PPK pistol found in his possession. Intelligence confirmed that O'Brien had been a PIRA 'volunteer' since 1992. He'd been active in London for several years and was suspected of planting a similar device earlier in the year which had been deactivated after failing to detonate. A list of other potential London targets was attributed to him.

The driver of the bus was ex-British army and had survived two postings in Northern Ireland unscathed. He sustained severe injuries in the explosion and became permanently deaf as a result. Another Irishman injured in the explosion was placed under armed police guard at the hospital for a couple of days because it was originally believed that he might have been O'Brien's minder.

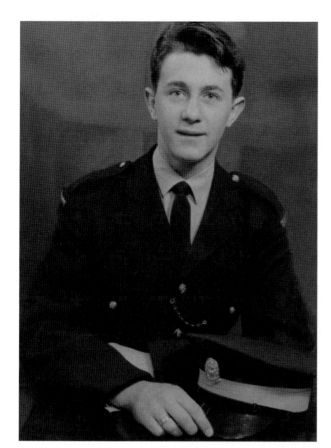

Ron Turnbull as a Fife
Police Cadet aged 17.

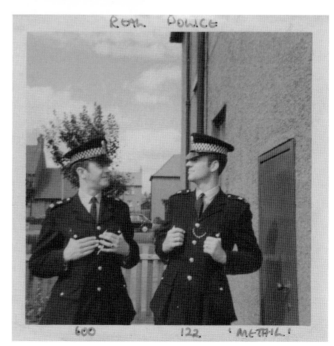

PCs Ron Turnbull
(left) and John Muir
during their time in
Fife Constabulary.

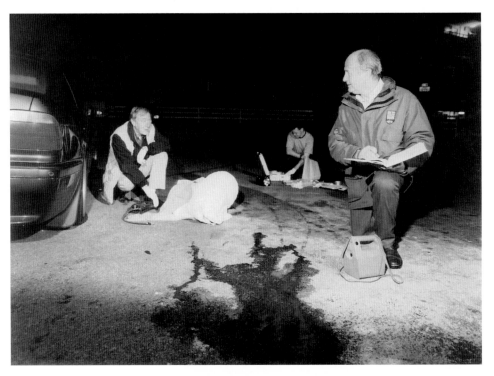

Ron Turnbull (right) and SOCO colleagues examining a shooting murder scene in south London 2002.

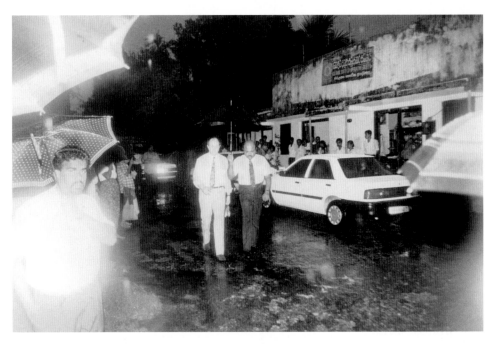

Ron Turnbull (left) with local police DCI (holding umbrella) at murder scene of politician in Sri Lanka 1993.

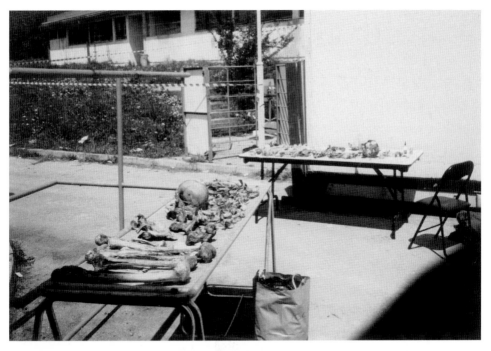

Skeletal reconstruction at Kalesija, Bosnia 1996.

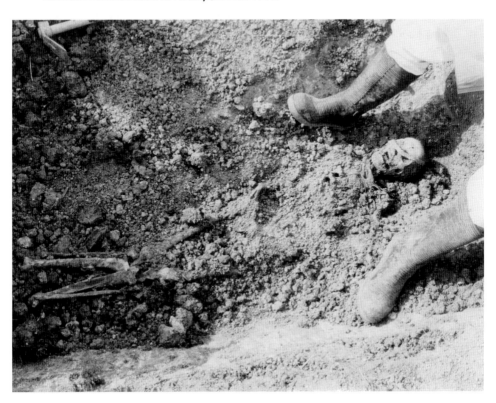

Victim of genocide in a mass grave, Kosovo 1999 (note the blindfold).

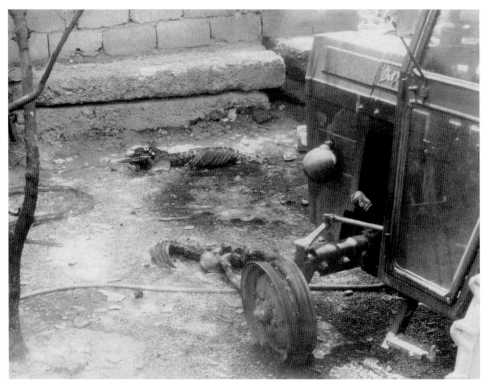

Burned bodies in compound of mass shooting in Celina village, Kosovo 1999.

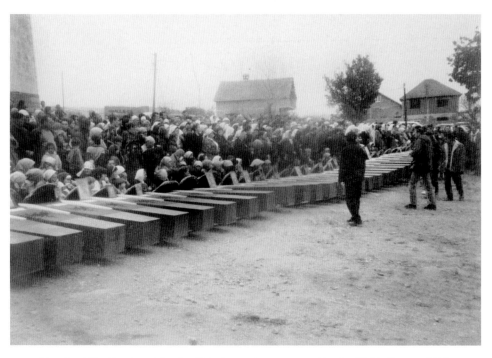

Mass burial by friends and family of Muslim victims recovered by the BFT in Kosovo 1999.

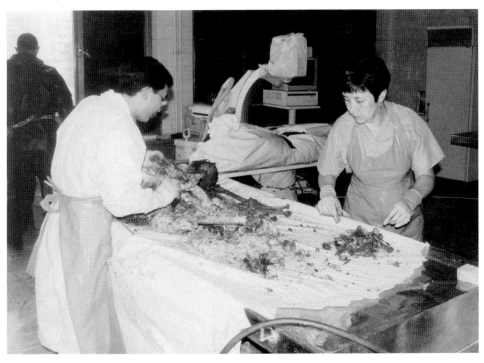

BFT autopsy and skeletal reconstruction in Pristina Hospital, Kosovo 2000.

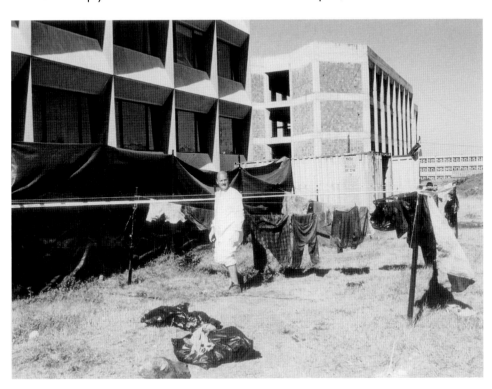

Mick Clarke on victims' clothes-cleaning duties at Pristina Hospital, Kosovo 2000.

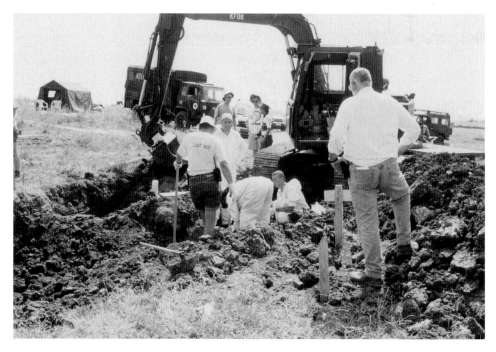

Ron Turnbull (left) with SIO Watts (right) and BFT colleagues at Dragonara cemetery Pristina, Kosovo 2000.

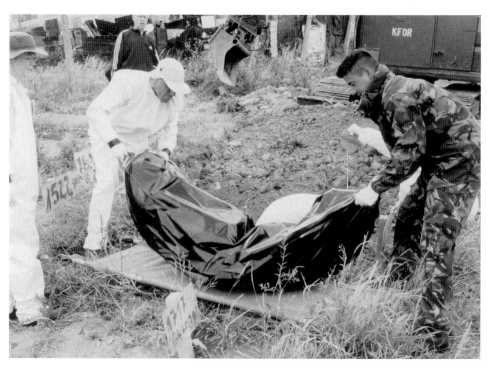

BFT and Royal Marine medic transporting body bag from Dragonara cemetery to Pristina hospital for autopsy, Kosovo 2000.

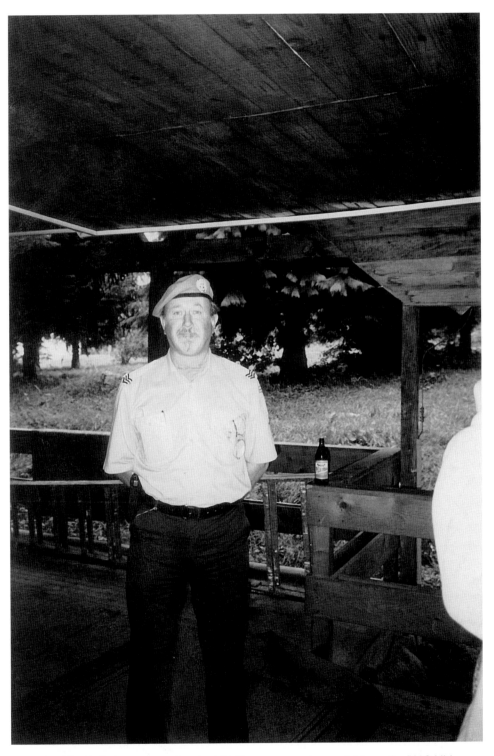

Ron Turnbull about to receive the UN Kosovo campaign medal from the RUC UN Police Commissioner in Kosovo 2000.

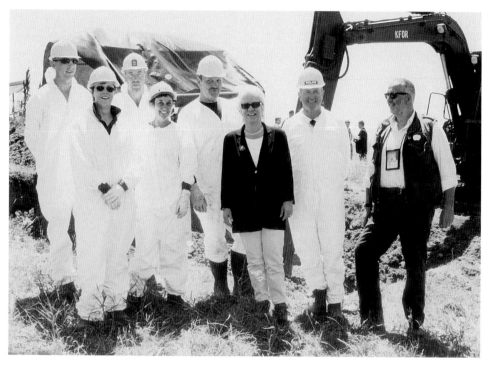

Ron Turnbull (2nd from right) with BFT colleagues and SIO Watts (right) during the visit of ICTY Chief Prosecutor Judge Carla del Ponti from The Hague at Dragonara cemetery, Pristina, Kosovo 2000.

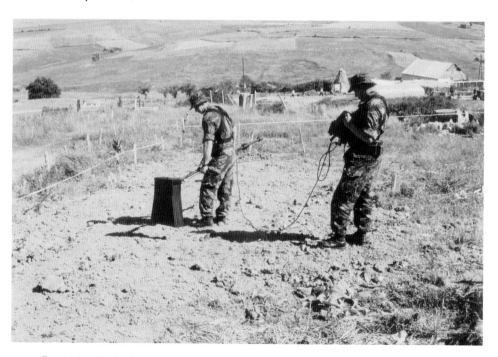

De-mining by the Norwegian army, Kosovo 2000.

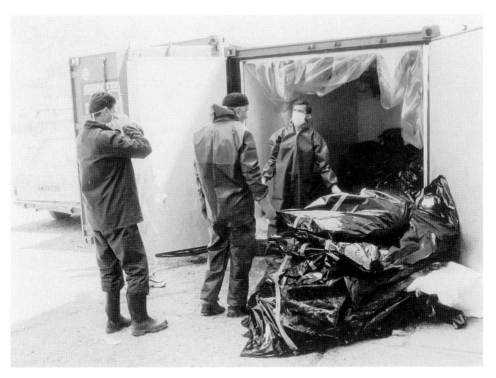

Body bags containing victims recovered by the BFT being removed by hospital staff from a refrigerated container for autopsy by BFT mortuary staff, Kosovo 2000.

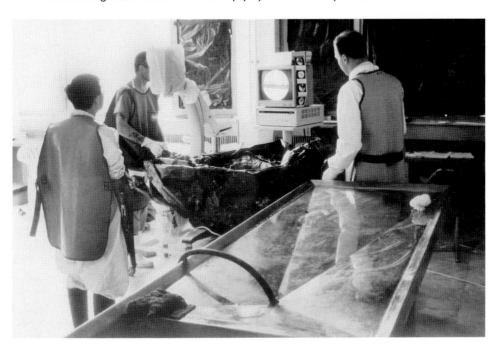

Fluoroscope examination of a body to determine the presence of metal during an autopsy in Pristina Hospital, Kosovo 2000.

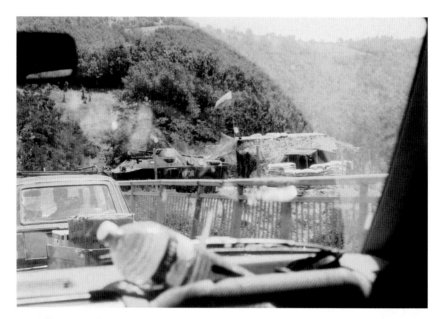

Polish military checkpoint soon after the BFT kidnap ordeal en route to Prizren, Kosovo 1999.

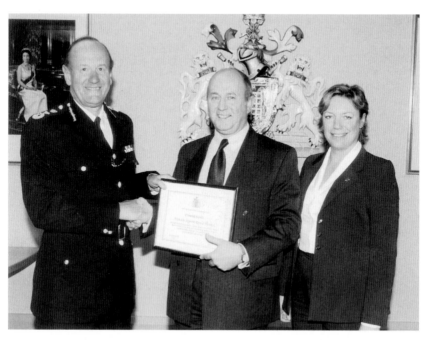

Ron Turnbull with wife Sheila receiving Commissioner's High Commendation from Sir John Stevens at NSY in 1999.

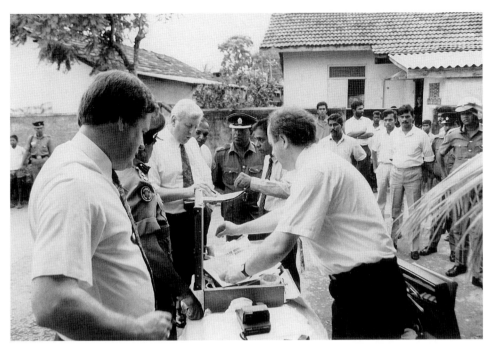

Ron Turnbull securing exhibits in murder bags at the scene of a political assassination in Sri Lanka 1993 while SIO Edwards briefs senior Sri Lankan police officers.

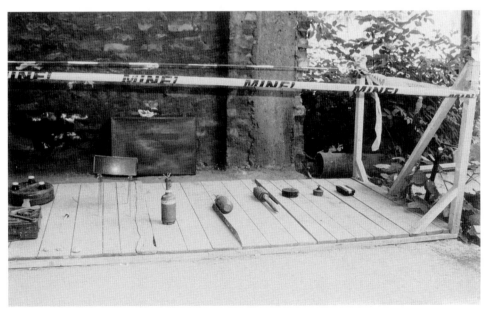

Land-mine awareness safety instruction module in Prizren, Kosovo 1999.

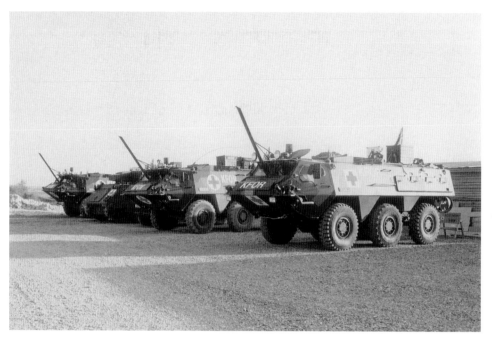

Norwegian army armoured personnel carriers (APCs) used for the safeguard of the BFT in Kosovo 2000.

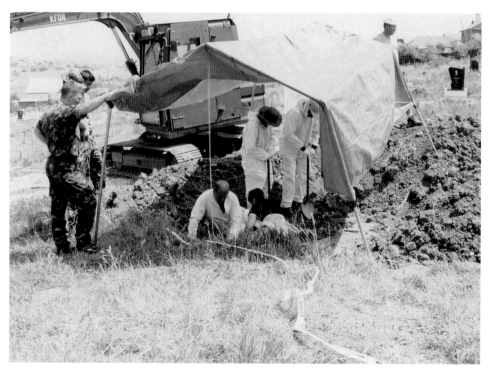

BFT exhumation in Dragonara cemetery, Pristina, Kosovo 2000 (Ron Turnbull on right of gazebo).

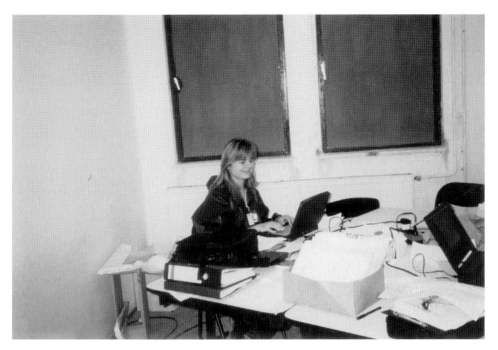

US pathologist Dr Milewski compiling the autopsy reports for PHR in Kalesija mortuary, Bosnia 1996.

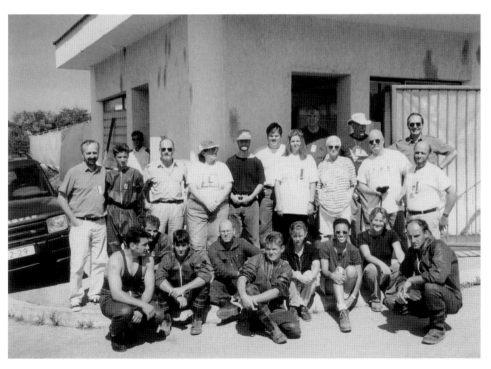

PHR staff at a temporary mortuary in Kalesija, Bosnia 1996 (Ron Turnbull in uniform and shades standing 3rd from left and Robert McNeill standing 3rd from right).

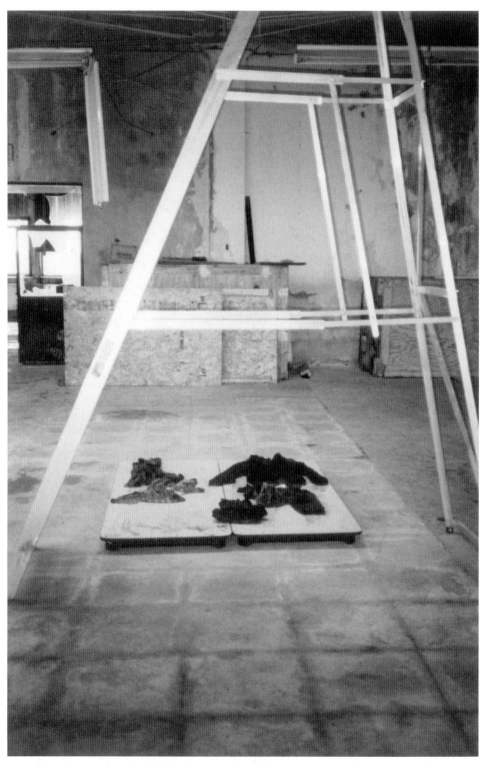

Photographing/recording victim's clothing in PHR mortuary Kalesija, Bosnia 1996.

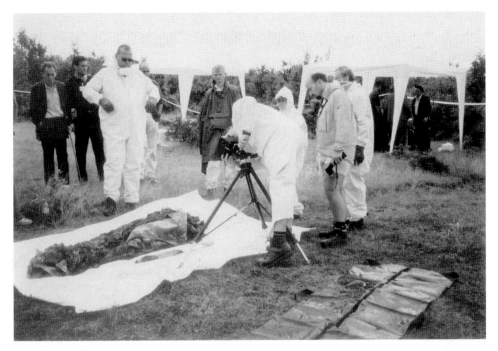

BFT staff processing exhumations in Kosovo 1999.

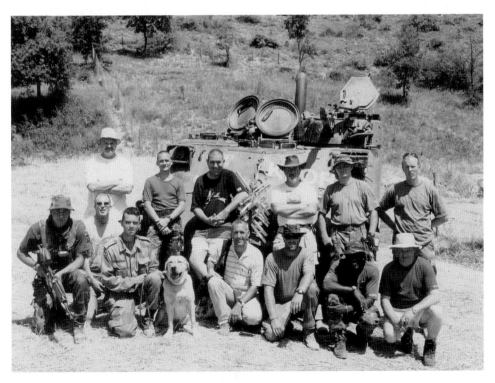

Forward site group of BFT colleagues with Norwegian army protection force in Kosovo 2000 (Ron Turnbull standing 3rd from right in hat).

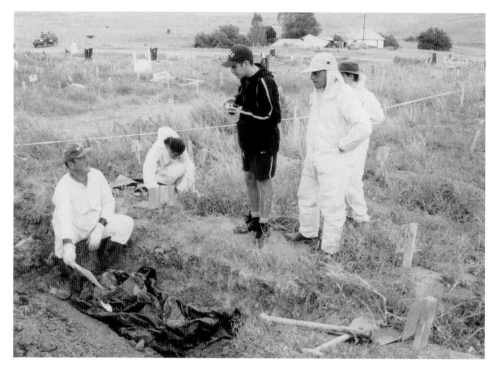

BFT staff photographing an exhumed body in Dragonara cemetery, Pristina, Kosovo 2000.

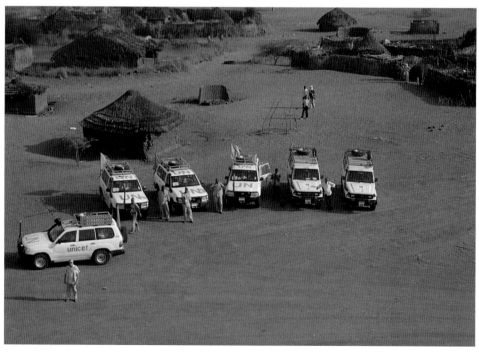

Ron Turnbull (extreme left) on a UNICEF/WFP security mission in Darfur, Sudan.

Chapter 26

Bosnia Calling

'The only thing necessary for the triumph of evil is for good men to do nothing.'

Edmund Burke (1729–97)
Philosopher & Politician

Four months later in July 1996 I was contacted by a prominent Home Office criminal pathologist with whom I'd carried out many post mortems who had just returned from war crime investigations in Bosnia and Herzegovina. He wanted to know if the Met would consider despatching an LLO to help set up legally acceptable scene of crime protocols in relation to exhumations and post-mortem examinations on hundreds of victims of war crimes and genocide. Initial investigations were being conducted there because of the war in Yugoslavia by a Boston-based medical humanitarian agency known as Physicians for Human Rights (PHR). PHR sought expert aid in evidence retrieval procedures that would be acceptable in a European criminal court in future prosecutions of war criminals. After much deliberation, briefings at the FCO and with the permission of the commissioner, I volunteered for this vitally important task. PHR had recently commenced work on massacre sites identified by witness testimony and NATO intelligence in the Srebrenica region.

PHR's team consisted of experienced medical personnel, forensic anthropologists (anthros), archaeologists (archaes) and criminal pathologists, supported by specialist technicians from the US, Central America, Europe and Scandinavia who because of their expertise were regularly called upon to respond to humanitarian disasters and atrocities in many parts of the world. I was soon flown to Zagreb, the capital of Croatia, spending most of the flight reading up on factors preceding the recent war in Yugoslavia, as well as trying to establish in my mind what I would require logistically for the task ahead. I met other members of the PHR team as we spent the night in a Zagreb hotel discussing the challenges and solution options we envisaged ahead of us. The following day we were convoyed to a town called Tuzla in Bosnia, after a detailed general security briefing. More data on the work that awaited us was disseminated while we consumed a packed lunch en route. The convoy consisted of white UN mini-buses driven by civilian police officers from various countries, seconded to aid their Bosnian colleagues, with lightly-armed US military vehicles as escort. Upon leaving beautiful Croatia via a military pontoon ferry pushed slowly and incredibly by an old tug across the Sava River because the only road bridge had been destroyed during the fighting, the horror of the conflict began to show in the drabness of the region on the Bosnian side of the river.

The destruction and desolation that we saw and the gaunt, almost distant look on the faces of people we passed on the troublesome roads, pot-holed by artillery fire, was alarming. There were no animals to be seen in the lush green fields, which struck me as odd. This was a slow, nightmarish journey through many military check-points manned by young, bored-looking soldiers in heavily-armed and sandbagged positions, some with battle tanks dug in around them. Helicopter gunships were seen and heard clattering around in the skies above.

When we eventually reached the town of Tuzla we were allocated various 'safe houses' and introduced to the two team leaders, both of whom were US medical doctors: one – an experienced and distinguished archaeologist from Seattle named Bill Haglund, who had operated for PHR in Rwanda, Guatemala and South America – was in charge of personnel at the grave sites; the other – an ex-Chief Medical Examiner for the city of Chicago – was in charge of the mortuary team, in which I would play a part. Bill had just completed an archaeological examination on the site of Custer's Last Stand at the Battle of Little Bighorn on behalf of the US army which fascinated us all as he kindly shared his notes with us over our joint evening meals. This boosted our morale greatly after long and grisly days dealing with numerous decomposing dead bodies.

Another team member for a short period was an American archaeologist who had recently returned from Burma (Myanmar) where social anthros had located an almost unknown tribe in the mountains there and found, to their surprise, that they were using crude aluminium implements and cooking pots. Tribespeople led the anthros to the source of these metal items which turned out to be part of a tail wing of a USAF airplane. The US army called in our colleague who retrieved the skeleton of the pilot deeply embedded in the hillside, still within the cockpit. It was a U-2 spy plane lost in combat, apparently. The pilot's remains were repatriated to the US and in the presence of his proud family rightfully buried with full military honours. What a fantastic operation to be part of. What splendid experts I had to work with and learn from.

The safe houses were large and multi-roomed but none had running water during daylight hours so we were obliged to set up a roster to ensure that a designated team member would arise at 0300 hours each day to fill the bath and all available receptacles with cold water which only ran between then and 0500 hours most mornings. Flushing of the toilets was restricted. We got used to the all-too-frequent bursts of 'happy fire' during weddings, birthdays or frankly any other festivities. Local men fired their AK-47 Kalashnikov rifles into the air as a form of celebration on these occasions. After a short local security briefing, we learned that we were resident and would operate in an American military zone of protection. We got accustomed to seeing GIs everywhere; for me, as one of the few Brits, this was an alien environment. Snipers were not entirely ruled out, we were told, but the main problems were land mines and unexploded ordnance. To walk outside of marked areas was out of the question. We were advised not to go anywhere alone, especially our female colleagues, and to wear UN caps or berets where possible in potentially 'hostile areas'.

Early the following morning, under the protection of the US army we travelled in an armed convoy to a bombed-out clothing factory in the small town of Kalesija to set up a temporary mortuary. This was to become almost a daily ritual. Miraculously UN engineers had installed solar-heated showers at this facility so that we could bathe after each day's mortuary work. This was an absolute luxury. We were informed of mass graves identified to the NATO forces by survivor and witness testimony which had been under military guard and were to be excavated on behalf of the ICTY in The Hague, Netherlands. Allegedly, near the end of hostilities Bosnian Muslim men had been bussed there from detention camps, then shot and buried in mass graves (see photo plate section).

I was given the formidable task of organizing an evidence retrieval system. I was shown artefacts retrieved from a site, but noted there was no formal record of when, where, or by whom they had been recovered. In other words, no chain of evidence custody was present which is essential for criminal court purposes. I'd brought along Met police self-seal, see-through exhibit bags in which I placed these items and began a chronological log to establish their validity. I unpacked my field kit and consumables and began preparing a shopping list of future requirements. At this time I was introduced to a Dutch police sergeant named Frank Frik who was a photographer and a former US auxiliary cop named Tim. Tim had been medically discharged in his first year of service with New Jersey Police after a shooting incident in which his issue shotgun was displaced from the rack within his police cruiser when a car crashed into the rear of his vehicle as he stopped to assist a fellow officer carrying out a traffic stop. This dislodgement caused the weapon to discharge, sending 12-gauge shot ricocheting around his cruiser injuring him in the neck and back and permanently damaging his hearing. Both these men were invaluable in setting up the evidence format with me. The rest of the team soon nicknamed us the 'Evidence Boys' or EBs. We set up procedures that became the UN's basic template for such missions in other parts of Bosnia and later on also in Kosovo.

One morning during breakfast in House No. 1 (there were two of them), an old TV that stood on top of a chest of drawers opposite the table at which we regularly ate crackled into life. It had obviously been left switched on for some time when there were no broadcasts. The RAF had blown up most aerial receivers during the war. As we heard this appliance crackling, we saw on the black and white screen a cartoon emerge which I identified as Noddy (with Bosnian subtitles). As the only Brit present it was truly comical as I tried to explain to the mainly American colleagues around the table who Noddy was. The fact that he lived with a guy called Big Ears didn't help, nor did the bells in their headgear. I was asked if they were gay, as if I'd know or care for that matter. Still, it made for a different and light-hearted start to our normal day.

My room-mate was a Swiss mortician who played saxophone rather well and who as a younger man had represented his country as an Olympic boxer. We had no facilities to phone home and speak with loved ones at first because the war had severely damaged the international telephone lines. Eventually engineers repaired them and so the international phone booths within the main Tuzla Post Office were available for use. Basically you entered a private booth, having told the staff which country you wished to connect with. They would hand you a slip of paper displaying that country's international code. Inside the glass booth there was a seat, a telephone and a large clock to let you know how long you would be on the line. I sat down and phoned my family, but could see that my Swiss pal in the opposite booth was having a bit of trouble. He would speak for a few seconds, then put the receiver down and repeat the process a couple of times, looking rather frustrated. When I finished my conversations I paid the counter staff – damn expensive it was too – and met up with him outside. I asked if all was well, but he told me he couldn't get through to his mother. A woman with a strange English sort of accent had answered the phone. He checked his mother's number, confirmed that it was correct, and rang again. Same result. Repeating the process for a third time, the same lady told him to stop annoying her. I asked to see the slip of paper he had been given and we both had to laugh. It bore the international code and country name of Swaziland. My buddy had been chatting to a lady in Africa. When we returned to our accommodation and recounted the tale it brought a smile to everyone's face. That evening one of the more artistic of our number sketched a coat of arms incorporating a Zulu-type shield bearing the Swiss cross and crossed assegai spears with African wild animals on either side. My colleague hung it in our bedroom and happily answered to the nickname of 'Swazi' for the rest of the tour. Amusingly, a couple of years ago he traced me on Facebook using 'Swazi' as his tag.

Having seen newsreel coverage of the war in Yugoslavia and read newspaper articles describing the countless allegations of atrocities committed by the participants, I had endeavoured to try to find out why this awful war had occurred. What I learned helped my understanding but in no way was my knowledge definitive; rather I arrived at a simplistic synopsis of what events and circumstances helped bring these tragic circumstances to fruition.

The Balkan Peninsula became a mix of Slavic tribes over the centuries which, although sharing a common language, became culturally separate. The areas we now know as Croatia and Slovenia were Westernized, became mainly Catholic and were prosperous. Serbia, under Moorish/ Turkish rule, was mainly Orthodox Christian and Muslim and was considerably poorer than its neighbours. The Balkan Wars erupted, hence the beginning of awful legacies that smouldered thereafter. Atrocities of mass executions, torture, rape, systematic imprisonment and ethnic cleansing unfolded. Over the years Serbia had won many concessions and was now extremely powerful in the region. A wave of nationalism swept over the country, ending with the notorious assassination of Archduke Franz Ferdinand of Austria in 1914 in Sarajevo, Bosnia by Serb activist Gavrilo Princip, one of six assassins assigned to kill the archduke during his visit, assuming that his demise would help to remove the presence of the Austro-Hungarian Empire from Serbia. Within weeks, the Great War broke out. At the end of the carnage of that conflict, Yugoslavia was born with the hope of unity in the region but instead the Serbians once again held the most dominant positions in the army, police and civil and diplomatic corps. Even the kings were Serbian. Other ethnic groups fared worse than before and so terrorism returned with the all-too-familiar tit-for-tat killings.

During the Second World War the Nazis occupied Yugoslavia and were fiercely resisted by the Serbs. At one stage Nazi savagery culminated in 100 civilians being shot in reprisal for every German soldier killed during the vicious Serb guerrilla campaign. The Croats, however, welcomed and more than a few actually collaborated with their new masters, who they hoped would liberate them from the Serbian yoke. As a result, German occupying forces set up concentration camps where thousands of Serbs, Jews and Romany gypsies were incarcerated and slaughtered with such brutality that records show even some Nazi officers considered this horrific. Memories of that holocaust remain vivid in the consciousness even to this day and many recall stories of that period when relatives were hacked or shot to death, burned alive in church buildings or dumped into mass graves in and outside of the death camps. The Croats also suffered terribly after the Second World War when the Serbs extracted revenge for their (Croat) collaboration with the Nazis.

President Josip Broz Tito emerged as Yugoslavia's communist leader at the cessation of the war. Although born a Croat, he intended to unite the nation. Remarkably he decided not to cause any investigations into the many internecine atrocities committed during the war, 'fearing this would only re-ignite the hatred festering between his people'. Instead he took the opposite course and forcibly suppressed all discussion and books etc. connected to same. Libraries and publishers were raided by his secret police and even private citizens' diaries and photographs were confiscated. After Tito's death in 1980 'collective presidencies' took over, which were seen to embody the principles of representing all regions and all ethnic groups. This appeared to last until 1989, albeit not too successfully, when Serb nationalism was again whipped up by politicians seeking supreme power. Serbian troops were sent to an Albanian Muslim region to allegedly 'liberate and protect the Serbian minority being persecuted there'. Shades of Nazi-ism? The autonomy of that region was removed and the Albanian university and schools closed. Serb police replaced local officers. These actions terrified Bosnians, Croats and others who feared a brutal return to old-style repression. Nationalism was stirred up everywhere as each group returned to its origins. The Soviet Union was collapsing at this time as well. The US and Europe became concerned that even more instability could escalate in the region and were horrified at the thought of Yugoslavia splitting up. Nationalist Serbs mistakenly believed that they would be the only country in the region supported by the military might of these participants in any armed struggle. Slovenia and Croatia declared independence in 1991 and Bosnia followed in 1992. Bosnia, with its mixed population of Serbs, Croats and Muslims quickly became the major battlefield as the Serb-controlled Yugoslav Army (JNA) sent tons of munitions and thousands of troops to 'support' Serbians there.

Chapter 27

The Village of Cerska in Bosnia and Herzegovina

I had my first intriguing insight into PHR field operations as I travelled to a site near the village of Cerska in the Srebrenica region which had been the centre of extremely hostile fighting. We passed through small homesteads that had been systematically and dramatically imploded, reducing them to rubble. Nearly all the properties in this region were fuelled by bottled gas. Apparently those responsible for this carnage lit candles in the basements, switched on all gas appliances and left the combination of gas and flame to do the rest, sometimes with the residents either unconscious, dead, or unbelievably still alive but trapped inside. Some outbuildings remained standing and bore proof of artillery and small-arms fire that had peppered the walls. Anything constructed of wood had burned. Shockingly obvious, however, and a vivid reminder of the ethnic cleansing that had occurred here, was the existence of recognizable national Serbian Orthodox Church insignia daubed in paint on several houses that stood relatively undamaged. Evidence that as the Serbian paramilitary forces came through this area they did not fire on friendly properties.

The grave site was under US military guard. It was agreed to de-mine it, then move in necessary equipment: e.g. sleeping containers that housed three or four bunk beds, portable toilets, generators, lighting and tarpaulins, as well as archaeological digging, removal and recording apparatus and as much clean water as could be transported. During the working day the military cordoned off the area with light tanks, 'Humvees' and Jeeps, a bizarre but reassuring sight in these still potentially dangerous locations where the local population did not always wish the evidence of their ethnic group's activities to be discovered. When night approached the field team withdrew, leaving the military encamped on site on guard; the most secure crime scene preservation I've ever experienced.

The site revealed standard evidence of this type of occurrence; interruption of the soil and irregular growing patterns of plants, for example. An initial perimeter search of the surface of this grave revealed clusters of 7.62mm cartridges of the type used in Kalashnikov AK-47 automatic rifles, indicating lines of fire. Bullet scorings were detected on trees opposite. Initial trial ditch excavations revealed disturbance of soil levels and some discolouration was evident as well as the presence of unidentified fluids. All of these factors also helped determine the potential size of the grave. Heavy plant such as trucks and/or bulldozers had left tracks here. Soil removals exposed boxes of shoes, then further excavation revealed skeletal remains. Intelligence led us to expect that all of the victims would be Muslim males, none of whom were military personnel.

Detailed mapping, sketching, video and photographic recording were all undertaken as attempts to differentiate the bodies began. This is extremely physically and emotionally exhausting work. As clearance progressed it was evident that layers of bodies were contained to a depth of several metres. Most were co-mingled, bore signs of trauma and firearm entry and exit wounds were commonplace. Disturbingly, most occupants were blindfolded or gagged and had their wrists and sometimes ankles crudely bound with wire, barbed wire on occasions.

The adult human skeleton consists of 206 bones and it is to the great credit of the anthros that most bones from each cadaver were recovered and placed in a marked body bag, each bag given a unique reference, e.g. CSK1, to denote the site and number of the cadaver. A flag marker displaying this number was photographed and mapped on the sketch plan. Before being sealed, any objects such as watches, bullets, cigarette lighters and tobacco tins, all of which were very common and which were considered to relate to a specific body were separately sealed in an evidence bag and placed within the relative body bag, which was then carefully and respectfully placed into a large refrigerated vehicle for transportation to the mortuary for autopsy.

Nothing prepares you for mass grave exhumation, no matter what experience you have. The sheer numbers can at first sight be almost overwhelming, so it's important for the co-ordinator to devise a pecking order and then ensure that all parties adhere to it. Normally this works well. Those not immediately engaged in the video or still photography and ground-penetrating radar (GPR) recording would check their equipment and discuss how they intended to progress when their time came to participate. Once the surface is recorded thus and evidence collected, the backhoe (mechanical excavator with a hinged bucket) starts the dig. This is a slow procedure with the operator under the supervision of an anthropologist, archaeologist, or oft times yours truly. As artefacts are exposed, the operator is asked to comb the floor of the dig extremely lightly with the edge of the bucket so that no body parts are damaged or lost. This takes experience and good handling skills by the operator. Once bones are confirmed, the backhoe pulls back and the experts step into the grave with their mattocks, picks and trowels to uncover the complete body. It is at this point when the true horror and barbarism hits home.

A feeling of great satisfaction came over us when an identifiable item was discovered. It was obvious that these men had been systematically searched by their killers so most sources of identification had been removed and probably destroyed. Photographs, receipts, certificates stating that the bearer was not fit for military service, ration books, etc. were recovered. As EBs cleaned, dried and carefully teased these items open, then with the aid of our translators, identified them, there was a noticeable 'buzz' at the evidence tables as colleagues congregated to see for themselves. We were in possession of a list of missing persons compiled by the ICTY to which we would refer at these times and we were able on several occasions to identify and pinpoint the region and/or village of the person listed.

I specifically recall finding a crumpled photograph in the wallet of a victim showing a young woman and two little girls, all in traditional costume, smiling towards the camera from a sunny garden. It was wrapped inside a child's crayoned drawing of a house and family. Two bullet holes had ripped through it. As I teased the photo out on to a drying board using water, scalpel and tweezers I became aware of a couple of female members of the team looking over my shoulder with tears in their eyes. I think the final insult of this cherished possession going to the grave with the father or other loved one of these little girls and probably their mother being destroyed by the murderer's bullet and thus preventing identification aroused emotions experienced and no doubt suppressed by all of us. Although we thought we'd hardened to our grisly task, every now and then something like this brought our hidden feelings to the fore. On these occasions we generally quietly downed tools and took a coffee or smoke break outside to grab a bit of fresh air and solitude while we individually gathered our thoughts before returning to our extremely vital tasks.

We uncovered many small cloth or leather pouches about 1in square, some ornately sewn, sealed and attached to leather thongs for wearing around the neck, or other times simply sewn into the hems of undergarments. We discovered that they contained handwritten Islamic prayers similar to tiny Christian bibles that can be worn on a charm bracelet; these were known as Muscas. They'd been written by local imams at the request of the head of a family and were worn to bring good fortune and protection. Where the imams were still alive, this could be a vital piece of evidence which was the case in several identifications. All unidentifiable Muscas were returned to Islamic leaders at the conclusion of enquiries for them to deal with as per the rules of their religion. Our translators told us that many of these unfortunate victims had been held in concentration camps for several years and had to make do with whatever materials they could find in order to survive the incredibly cold winters. It became the habit of women relatives of these incarcerated men to sew such items into the linings or hems of their menfolk's jackets or coats when they knew that occupying forces were approaching and the likelihood that their loved ones would be arrested and interred, or even much worse, in the hope that it may identify them in the future.

Smoking utensils were found on or near almost every body. These generally took the shape of clay pipes, cigarette papers, loose tobacco and many small tins containing flints and stones. Some were inscribed with names which were of interest and useful to us. Small waxed bags of dried fruit and sugar were commonplace, occasionally wrapped in embroidered handkerchiefs bearing female names or just initials. A few promissory notes written by community leaders were found, guaranteeing money for the safe passage of the bearer or to reward good treatment while in detention. We later learned from the writers of such notes that they had been told by the captors of these men when being taken to work camps that such notes were 'To aid in rebuilding the country at the cessation of hostilities.'

A full post-mortem examination was carried out on each cadaver and evidence of physical torture, treated and untreated wounds as well as the presence of ballistic or other evidential artefacts in each body was recorded, retrieved and a cause of death sought. Not all bodies gave signs of being shot. In such cases, where only skeletal remains existed, a cause of death was not established, although bullets may have passed through the body causing death without leaving a trace. Gruesomely, it isn't feasible that all were in fact dead when the grave was filled in. Some may have been injured or rendered unconscious and tragically suffocated to death, again leaving no trace. Some bodies retained human tissue in an advanced state of adipocerous decomposition which did not help physical recovery or the post-mortem examination. In this condition, the soft tissues are reduced to a fatty, waxy, soap-like consistency which is not agreeable to the nostrils. A great deal of evidence existed of multiple shootings in which several different calibres of bullets were recovered. Post-mortem examinations of 154 bodies in this one grave retrieved 1,230 bullets which were sent to the FBI Lab in Quantico, USA for potential ballistic comparison against any recovered weapons.

The task of the anthropologist was primarily to assist pathologists in determining the cause of death but also, and equally important, to establish sex, probable age and assist with identification. Any apparent physical abnormality in bones such as limps or pronounced jaw disfigurements would be of great assistance. However, problems were encountered from the outset. Only one or two of the bodies showed evidence of having had dental work. We knew that these poor souls were of peasant stock and there was little or no dentistry in the region from where they came, emergency hospital extractions apart. Consequently no dental records, which are a standard standby, were available. Hospitals had also been targeted by the invaders and many were reduced to rubble and medical records destroyed.

International pathologists plus their technicians worked closely with the evidence team (EBs). We recorded the removal of each body bag from a refrigerated vehicle, then accompanied it to the X-ray fluoroscope facility where it was opened and the contents photographed. The pathologist would then identify and remove any accessible bullets, fragments or wire bindings highlighted by the X-ray device and record same in the autopsy report, adding their initials and number; thus a bullet from CSK1 became CSK1/1/YIM, for example. These items were taken to the evidence area and fully examined, recorded and cleaned. Any identifiable items of clothing were removed, recorded and photographed with the intention of identifying the wearer. Under the strict control of other anthropologists, the deceased's clothing was cleaned on site by anthropology students in case small bones or other items of evidential value were entangled, ably assisted by locally-recruited former Bosnian soldiers. A system of sieve traps was devised just outside the factory building to ensure that nothing was lost in a rather Heath Robinson conveyor-belt system installed by the highly-inventive PHR engineers. As water was still not on tap, we had to rely on military tankers bringing it to us. We had to ensure that at the end of each day we had enough water left to shower in after rationing it to the body and clothes cleaning teams who were by now referred to as the 'bone-washers'.

I recall one of the bone-washers saying: 'The bodies wear their clothes like shrouds.' This seemed to aptly voice what most of us were feeling. The wet clothing was hung out on washing lines and eventually shown to relatives after we learned that clothing was a vital aid to identification, therefore we placed more emphasis upon it than normal. Open days were held so that all who wanted to view this clothing for ID purposes could do so. This was very successful on a number of levels, so much so that it was continued in later sites I was involved with in Kosovo.

We discovered individuals dressed in home-made garments created out of military parachute material, some patched with curtain material. One tragic individual had electrical duct tape wrapped around his stockinged feet in lieu of any more robust footwear. Some of these unfortunate souls had been held in concentration camps for several years and had to make do with whatever clothing material they could find in order to survive the severity of a Balkan winter. As much detail as possible was gleaned from each cadaver, photographed and compiled into a directory (album) beside a physical description of the body. This was shown to relatives in the hope of identification and I'm glad to say was successful in a number of cases.

During PHR's spell in Kalesija many women bussed to Tuzla from the Srebrenica region became aware of our work. A deputation, accompanied by a local film crew, was permitted access to the facility so that we could explain the procedures we were undertaking and confirm to them that the bodies of their kinsmen were being treated properly and with total respect. I recall a letter being read out by one such lady from a grieving relative who asked: 'Can I be given a small bone so that I can carry it and sleep on it until I get my son's body back?' Obviously this could not be permitted, but it demonstrated the intensity of the women's grief and instilled in us even more determination to find evidence against the cruel perpetrators of these atrocities, as if any more was required.

Chapter 28

Vukovar Hospital in Croatia

The next site on PHR's list involved victims from Vukovar Hospital, Croatia, known as Ocvara Farm, which lay some 10 kilometres south of Vukovar, near the village of Grabovo. Intelligence revealed that patients, doctors, nurses, Red Crescent workers and even menial hospital staff had been taken away, killed and buried in a mass grave when Serbian forces overran it. Of the 300 men known to be alive at the end of hostilities being treated in this hospital, 261 were missing, believed dead. This figure does not include medical personnel. This atrocity was carried out after UN military observers were permitted by senior personnel of the occupying Yugoslav army (JNA) to visit the hospital, but before armed UN peacekeepers could liberate and protect it. The hospital was then under the joint command of JNA and Serbian paramilitary troops. The mass grave site was similar to the Cerska site and we dealt with it in a similar manner. However, in this site female bodies would also be discovered.

The normal European database which anthros rely upon to gauge the estimation of age of skeletal remains had to be abandoned due to the fact that the physical state of the bone structure of many of these bodies was far more retarded than expected. Some teenage boys' skeletons were prematurely stunted and their spines bent, indicating that they had carried out extremely heavy manual work from a very early age, probably lifting and carrying heavy weights on their shoulders or heads for lengthy periods. It was known that such peasant agricultural work was arduous because it was not aided by modern machinery found in other parts of Europe. Forestry, logging and mining were also routine tasks carried out in the open in all weathers, with such workers often dressed in inadequate or scant clothing. Added to this were a poor and under-nourishing diet, poverty and lack of medical treatment which complicated the estimation even further. To compensate for this, the overall skeleton, skull and pubic symphysis (joint formed by the hip bones situated just above the crotch) were examined in finer detail than usual.

The skull, and pelvic or innominate bones (such as the hip bone), were vital in determining sex. The skull can also be of use in determining racial origin but this was not an issue here. Detailed examination of the scapulae was also carried out in order to form an opinion as to the left- or right-handedness of the body as well as to assist with an age guesstimate. Yet again, poor bone structure made this more difficult so broader than normal percentages for error were put in place. Any ballistic trauma evident in the skeleton was calibrated in detail and photographed. At the conclusion of the post-mortem process samples of the long bones were taken coupled with selected molars where applicable and were forwarded to a European lab to be stored for comparison with parental or familial DNA samples that might be taken for identification purposes in the future.

A familiar pattern in ethnic cleansing atrocities is the targeting of professionals, academics and intelligentsia. There was indisputable proof in the former Yugoslavia that the medical profession was singled out for special treatment. Doctors and nurses who tended prisoners of war were also killed when the UN forces started to enforce the ceasefire and tried to regain control. Several hundred medics were missing from this hospital, presumed dead. These caring people must never be forgotten. They were not soldiers killed in combat. They must not be allowed to have died in vain, especially when evidence of their abhorrent and shameful demise is capable of proof and those responsible can and should be brought to justice. Only then can the former Yugoslavia work towards its own future.

The first time I visited Sarajevo was not for the best of reasons. A tragic accident had taken the life of a UN mine-clearance specialist in our employ plus his de-mining dog and a local man he was training. Several others were injured. A former Rhodesian army officer who led our mine-clearance staff knew that the Mines Advisory Group (MAG) had an office in Sarajevo that may be able to put us in touch with suitably-experienced candidates looking for such work in the region. We couldn't start new sites without these experts clearing them, so finding a replacement was vital and the sooner the better. We found the MAG office in a pretty shot-up part of the city. The expo obviously knew the guy who was sitting at the reception desk. As he introduced us I saw that he wore a black patch over his left eye, his left lower arm and hand were artificial and as he dragged a seat over for me, I noted his right leg was also false. Trying not to look too surprised, we talked business and he made a couple of phone calls that ended with us hiring another expo. We popped into The Harp public house near the football stadium for a spot of lunch. It was run by a former soldier of the Royal Irish Rifles Regiment. As we became more comfortable with one another I jokingly said to the MAG rep that it must have been one hell of an explosion that caused his injuries. He told me that in fact it had been two separate blasts. He'd been a Royal Navy diver who specialized in mine clearance. We all agreed over the last beer that he may not be the MAG's best advert for recruiting staff, but there was no-one else.

Nearing the end of my secondment I was again driving a UN Jeep through Sarajevo in the company of a colleague as we sought supplies. The area had suffered severely during the war and a lengthy siege with over 60 per cent of buildings destroyed or seriously damaged. As I drove towards the airport, where fighting had been at its peak, all around was rubble. The fronts of apartments had been blown away, leaving the contents, such as they were, in full view. Displaced families had occupied many of them, making shelters with tarpaulin, as smoke from open fires could be seen billowing upwards from these scant shelters. Artillery shells and thousands of bullet holes had pockmarked the walls. Smashed telegraph poles and lamp posts littered the carriageway where burned-out shells of trams, buses and cars lay abandoned in the road, some on their sides, and had to be negotiated slowly in order to pass by. Once attractive trees that lined the central reservation now stood charred and broken. Eerily, I didn't see or hear any birds. It could have been a scene from a *Mad Max* movie.

When I reached the bottom of a long hill I saw a US Texas Ranger police cruiser parked in a lay-by with the driver resplendent in his wide cowboy hat, sheriff-style badge and cowboy boots showing two local Bosnian policemen how to operate a radar speed gun. He waved as we passed by. Was this normal law enforcement returning to Sarajevo? I recall saying to my colleague: 'Speed traps, I ask you.' Ironically they were standing next to a poster that I'd seen many times and knew from one of our translators that it proclaimed in the Bosnian language 'Arm your Children'. Later that day as we walked through the old Moorish craft centre of Sarajevo in our UN Protection Force (UNPROFOR) uniforms, an elderly lady dressed sombrely in black approached us. She smiled, held out her hand, and as I took it she leaned up and placed a small red rose in my shirt pocket, kissed me on the cheek and said, 'Thank you UN, thank you sir.' As I stood there a little embarrassed, she smiled and walked off. Less charitable colleagues inferred that she was hoping for a payment for the flower, but I don't think so.

At the end of our enquiries all of the evidence obtained at Kalesija was handed over against signature to a UN legal representative and along with each pathologist's report transported to the ICTY in The Hague where I was soon once more instrumental in setting up protocols for other massacre and burial sites in the Balkans.

At this time there were still literally thousands of victims lying in mass graves in Bosnia alone. At least 150 such graves were known but not enough of them were under military protection. There were 2.7 million refugees and internally displaced persons. Between 2 and 6 million land mines were estimated to lie undetected and uncharted. Thousands of NATO troops kept the factions apart. Had it not been for their intervention, I doubt if peace would have lasted long. In 1996 only one low-ranking soldier had been convicted of war crimes attributable to Srebrenica. He received ten years' imprisonment. Those defending him tried to invoke the Nuremburg defence so often heard at the trials of Second World War Nazi war criminals. In other words, 'he was only acting under orders and refusal to comply would have resulted in his own immediate death at the hands of his officers.'

A few survivors of these mass murders who had escaped from trucks conveying them from concentration camps to be shot in this way gave different testimony. One had feigned death when the bullets of the killers missed him as he lay still in the grave alongside his dead friends. He overheard soldiers say that they couldn't be bothered to fill in the grave that night but would return in the morning to do so. He escaped when darkness fell. These lucky but brave witnesses told of 'drunken and noisy soldiers insulting and humiliating blindfolded and bound men who were kneeling before pre-dug gravesites as they opened up on them with their AK-47s. Officers laughing with them as they (the officers) fired their pistols into the back of the heads of some of them.' Definitely not the actions of soldiers acting under orders, I would submit. The latter of these witnesses was under armed police protection at an undisclosed location somewhere in Europe because he was a major witness in this prosecution and would probably repeat his testimony in the forthcoming trials of more senior war criminals, or at least I hope so.

Some fifty-seven persons had already been indicted by the ICTY on charges of war crimes including genocide, and many more would follow. So much was still to be done and I was damn sure I would be involved in as many of these investigations as possible. To say the least, I was so appalled and moved by what I had witnessed in Bosnia that I felt compelled to channel my efforts and lend my gained expertise to assist with war crime investigations in this region wherever possible. With the support of a number of forward-thinking senior Met officers and the authority of the FCO I was able to do so, returning on several occasions in 1997/8 to Bosnia, Kosovo and the Republic of Srpska to assist ICTY investigation teams in the forensic examination of other sites of war crimes, some of which resulted in the arrest of perpetrators. Intermittently I was also dealing with major crime investigations in my day job for Scotland Yard, both in the UK and former Commonwealth countries as and when required.

Chapter 29

The British Forensic Team: Kosovo 1999

In 1999 I was selected by the FCO and despatched as forensic co-ordinator with a senior member of that establishment and as SIO the supremely-experienced Commander John Bunn, QPM from Scotland Yard's Anti-Terrorist Squad, to set up the British Forensic Team (BFT) in Kosovo. We were based initially in Skopje, Macedonia, from where I obtained four 4x4 vehicles plus equipment and stores for our eventual move into Kosovo where we were to be embedded with a British army Royal Military Police (RMP) contingent heading for the capital city of Pristina. We entered that war-torn country as NATO troops were clearing the northern enclaves, but as there was still sporadic armed resistance the military decided it was too dangerous for our little group of unarmed civilians to continue with them so we were left in the very capable hands of the German military in the old Moorish former capital city of Prizren while the remainder of north Kosovo was stabilized. Prizren was a fascinating old city situated along the ancient spice route from the Middle East. We rented accommodation in a number of flats and were well looked after by our thankful Muslim hosts.

Over the following six months we recycled members of the BFT on a monthly basis, bringing in volunteers from the UK, Australia and the Netherlands as per an FCO rota. These were pathologists, forensic anthropologists, fluoroscope technicians, mortuary technicians, police photographers, police body recovery teams, SOCOs and detectives, as well as local interpreters to investigate more than fourteen separate sites of alleged massacre. We recovered 194 bodies in total, of which 160 were male, 15 female and 19 unknown due to skeletal disruption. Of these, 106 were identified and returned to their loved ones with the aid of ICTY investigators on the ground. In total this year, combined international exhumation teams (including the BFT) examined 146 sites where they recovered 1,785 bodies of which 893 were identified. This was a massive task carried out by dedicated personnel to the highest of standards and rightly earned the BFT a great deal of respect within the military and more especially with local communities, as well as from other national forensic teams so deployed.

Basically we split the BFT into two units. An SIO led the recovery team in the field after agreeing the venue with the ICTY and arranging all necessary security during travel and site protection. The recovered bodies were transported to refrigerated containers for post-mortem examination, normally the following day. That evening the SIO or myself would inform the mortuary team of the site history and numbers we'd collected and once the mortuary team began their work they would update us of the results of their findings on the cadavers we had brought in the day before. That way everyone knew what was happening and about to happen. It worked very well. Occasionally staff would interchange within the teams to give them an insight into the other unit's workings. Again this was a valuable asset as we rotated staff later on in the mission. The pathologists' findings and the SIOs' reports were jointly submitted to the ICTY for consideration of inclusion in any future criminal trials at the tribunal. A number of these reports were used in this way. It was most rewarding work.

We started by investigating some reasonably freshly dug areas and mounds of smashed buildings and rubbish that NATO troops had been told contained bodies of persons, mostly men, who had disappeared from various nearby villages. The reasons for this were threefold:

- The BFT needed to hone their excavation skills
- NATO wanted to release soldiers from guarding these sites for other more important tasks
- The ICTY had not finished preparing a list of confirmed burial sites.

What we uncovered initially were mainly carcases of farm animals that had probably fallen foul of artillery fire. Others were simply the remains of farm outbuildings that had suffered the same fate. Locals still insisted that their lost loved ones must therefore be underneath these carcases and rubbish, but we'd taken sufficient samples and dug deeper in case that was so. In one of these digs we uncovered a tarpaulin wrapped tightly around bulbous items. This turned out to be four paws from a large brown bear and a cabbage. We had no idea what that was about, although we knew that entertainers using dancing bears travelled around the region before hostilities began. Perhaps such a poor dancing bear had become someone's fodder?

One such site we referred to as the Red Dam as it was next to a reservoir used by a local aluminium factory at Karakaj (aka Benice Dam) which caused the water to turn a rusty red colour. Our protection force here was a Russian army paratrooper unit for the first and only time. They were impressive. Intel told us this had been a massacre site where lorryloads of men were driven, mainly during the hours of darkness, and shot in lines of about a dozen next to pre-dug trenches and then pushed into the void. Any victims still showing signs of life were despatched by an officer's handgun via a head shot. Another dozen would follow until the mound of human bodies nearly reached the surface, at which time lime was thrown in and a backhoe bulldozed the topsoil over them. A survivor who escaped having feigned death while the killers drank alcohol and failed to fill in a grave till the following morning told NATO that the executions took place between 14 and 15 July 1995 involving Muslim men from the nearby village of Bratunac. They'd been held in Petrovci School (2km from the dam) while the graves were being prepared. He overheard soldiers humiliating their bound captives as they pushed them to the graveside and, pointing at the dead bodies already in the grave, said 'Choose a free spot.'

Initial surface examination of this site revealed 1,030 shell cases on a plateau that was probably used as a firing point; 900 at ground level around the grave; 150 sounded by metal detector just under the surface; plus 38 small body parts; 3 items of ID (a bank card plus general correspondence); numerous Muslim artefacts and slip-on-style shoes favoured by Muslims; and interestingly, an automatic Seiko watch displaying the date 'Sun 16'.

From the numbers we were given that had allegedly been slaughtered here it seemed improbable that the single trench we had identified from aerial photography and a study of the vegetation plus geology held them all. However, as the backhoe reached the bottom of the grave, or so we thought, a test dig underneath this point threw up more artefacts and combing revealed the presence of wooden planks like railway sleepers. We brought in a larger backhoe, removed the planks and discovered another level of bodies. Backhoe tracks were visible, which we photographed in detail lest the excavator that had made these should ever be traced, then this lower pile of bodies was removed. Those responsible had dug down as far as their backhoe would allow, then formed a ramp with the sleepers allowing the backhoe to get further down into the grave and dig another of similar dimensions below it, alighting in the same way. We took a photographic record of the marks the bucket cuts had left in the soil (striation marks), again to compare these with any suspect bucket identified at a later stage.

The area around this site included a couple of Serbian enclaves, the occupants of which did not relish the BFT discovering evidence that may be used against their countrymen in The Hague court so it was decided that an initial security reconnaissance should be undertaken. The Russian military had set up a secure camp near to the dam, so with the O/I/C and a corporal in tow as translator we viewed the exact area where we would be working. At the top of the dam there stood a small brick hut that had obviously something to do with the maintenance of the reservoir and I asked if it had been cleared as it may attract squatters or even worse, I thought. The corporal informed me that they would send in a search team and clear it, which they did. It was empty. For the duration of our stay at that site they placed a sentry up there which gave us peace of mind, I can assure you. We had an APC on this site into which we could scramble should any hostile crowd appear. There had been veiled threats of this from locals at an early stage of negotiations. We'd only used an APC once earlier when youths formed a stone-throwing group and our protection force had us climb swiftly into it as they moved the stone-throwers away and extended and reinforced the outer cordon. Sitting inside this vehicle as stones noisily bounced off the exterior was not very pleasant, but of course it could have been a lot worse. The Russian soldiers also used us as unwitting participants in their 'stag' operations. Basically, without our knowledge and before our arrival some mornings, the NCOs would install sentries in various places of concealment where they would remain throughout the day as we worked on, oblivious to their presence. It was quite a surprise to us, myself included, when a small bush or grassy knoll stood up and a sniper in full camouflage gear walked off towards their camp after an NCO barked out an order. Undeniably great practice for the soldiers and quite reassuring, if not a trifle alarming and rather amusing for us.

I recall stepping back from the action at this site, watching what all my expert colleagues were doing and feeling proud of what we were accomplishing. These victims of the most horrific of atrocities had been savagely murdered by people who offered them no mercy and even less respect. They had been buried, and often dug up and re-buried as NATO forces drew near, by these cowards trying to cover up their awful deeds. Now we could hopefully give them a voice. I remember saying to a photographer colleague: 'Kosovo is two hours away by plane from the UK and not much longer by car down the autobahn from Germany. We fly over it going on holiday. How the hell did we let this happen?' Depraved psychopaths had booby-trapped graves and buildings, also inserting these abhorrent devices in children's toys in order to maim or kill more innocent victims. Snipers had shot children and the elderly as they collected water in such a way that they were severely injured but not killed in the hope that others would come to their assistance and be caught in the cross-hairs of their rifles. Diabolical to say the least.

I learned from our Russian hosts during an evening meal to which they treated us in their mess on our last day working with them that Robert Burns, Scotland's national bard, is a much-revered poet there. The Russian CO had a better knowledge of some of Burns' work than I did, to be fair, as he regaled me with a few verses during a vodka-toasting session after the meal was over.

The BFT was first of the international forensic teams in theatre and as others came on site I was asked by a senior ICTY investigator to address them before they were deployed to known sites throughout the country. I was happy to do so. During the presentation I made the audience aware of the mistakes we'd made in order to save them a lot of time, emphasized the need to include local villagers, most of whom would be relatives of the victims, and the sensitivities that we'd experienced with regard to different cultural needs. I went on to describe how the BFT carried out the process we had so far found to be the best use of resources and left it up to them to pick what they saw as positive and discard those aspects that they didn't require or could do better their way. At the end of my presentation these teams – who hailed from Austria, Belgium, Canada, Denmark, Finland, France, Germany and Spain plus a US FBI team – were split up to meet their respective ICTY investigators and to discuss the sites they would soon examine. As I shared a coffee with my ICTY colleague, we were approached by a member of the audience who identified himself as a Swiss forensic expert. A one-man team. The ICTY investigator asked him who he would like to work with, to which he replied that he had no preference. Asked what his mother tongue was he said he spoke several languages but primarily German and eventually chose to become part of the much smaller Austrian team.

A matter of considerable pride for me and the BFT was that ICTY investigators began to inform us that on many occasions as they made initial visits to villages to consider the possibility of conducting forensic investigations in their region, village leaders asked if the BFT could do it. Praise indeed.

There's absolutely no doubt in my mind that such involvement, whether it be in Bosnia, Kosovo or any other war-torn arena, changes and shapes you forever. Your daily involvement and experiences would be more than a put-off for most people. Yet the camaraderie shared with fellow experts from separate disciplines creates a bond like no other, and I include in that the very special bond shared by police officers in their day-to-day work, as evidenced by the friendships and support of many of these individuals that I still share to this day. I learned so much about my capabilities, my professionalism and especially about me as a person. The memories, thoughts, experiences and sadness of the Balkans will never leave me (see photo plate section).

Chapter 30

The Village of Celina in Kosovo

One of the crime scenes that made the biggest impression on me and all of the others in the BFT was in the village of Celina. Celina was a mainly Albanian (Muslim) village that had suffered badly during the war in Yugoslavia, mainly due to its known alliance, support and involvement with the Kosovan Liberation Army (KLA) who fought relentlessly against the Serbian forces. Geographically it lies on the main Prizren to Đakovo road near the villages of Krusha e Madhe and Velika Kruša in which we would be involved in even more gruesome body recovery as well. When NATO alliance military operations began in March 1999 it was hoped that killings would cease, but tragically this was not the case. In fact, they escalated as Serb paramilitaries swept through the area to remove any trace of their crimes. As the heavily-armoured units began to encircle these small villages the occupants, some 2,000 of them, fled. Those who didn't flee but hid in their cellars were burned in their homes. Others were shot in the open. Most were robbed of anything valuable which they offered up to their adversaries on the promise of being allowed to leave. As soon as the bounty was handed over the lucky ones were shot; others were locked in their cellars and burned alive. As a police officer I was appalled to hear from several survivors that local Serb policemen who were known to the villagers took part in these atrocities and robbed people they had known for years before killing them.

Personnel of the Organization for Security and Cooperation in Europe (OSCE) Kosovo Verification Mission, a security-oriented inter-governmental organization, had been in the region until 20 March. Over the following few days infants in their cots and an old man aged 106 were among those massacred. Children were killed in front of their parents, men before their wives and kids, under-age girls were raped in front of their families, heaps of shot men were soaked in petrol and set alight, after which the buildings were bulldozed not only to destroy any

176

evidence but also to deter anyone left alive from continued resistance or informing NATO forces. In total seventy-five Celina residents were butchered in this way (see photo plate section).

This became an all-too-familiar pattern for us as we moved from village to village. Similar tragic stories of inhuman atrocities, massacre, sexual deviation, depravation and almost unbelievable horror confronted us. It was BFT practice to sit with the elders of each village or those responsible for the area in which we would be operating in order to explain what our brief was, how we'd deal with their deceased loved ones and what our ultimate objective was, vis-à-vis the arrest of those responsible for these diabolical crimes. This was a slow process as everyone wanted to speak and tell us their horrific tale. We had to invoke a great deal of sympathy, diplomacy and patience in these meetings, but we got there. Ironically the BFT was approached by families not included in the ICTY brief to recover their loved ones. Normally we had to refuse such requests, but a couple of exceptions were made. It would be nigh on impossible to list every site covered by the BFT, so I hope that no individual or group is offended if they do not find any reference to a lost loved one from their village within these chapters.

As you would expect, there was a great deal of media interest in what the BFT was accomplishing, not only from UK newspapers and TV channels but from journalists and reporters worldwide. As the SIO, John dealt with the lion's share of these interviews so that the rest of the team could get on with their vital work. He also let it be known that after a given date no further interviews would be possible because they were seriously eating into his time and attention to team tasks. John returned to the UK for a short break, leaving yours truly to carry on the day-to-day teamwork.

Before leaving on this mission I'd spoken with my mother in Scotland, who was not in the best of health, telling her I would be away for a couple of months 'on a course in America'. I didn't want her to worry needlessly on my account if she knew I'd be in a war zone as this would not have helped her recuperation. During John's absence a member of our security cordon found me at the centre of an exhumation site and told me that a TV reporter wanted to speak to the SIO. I spoke with the reporter, who turned out to be representing China's national TV channel and who had only just obtained permission to travel to Kosovo. He requested an interview on camera to which I agreed after ascertaining that it would only be broadcast in the Chinese region. Unbeknown to me, the region of China included Australasia. You learn something new every day.

The father of one of my old school chums, Roy Nowicki, also a good friend of my mother, was visiting his daughter in Australia where he saw this interview on TV. On returning to Scotland he popped in and told my mum what he'd seen and described the role in which I was engaged. Mum then contacted my favourite cousin's ex-police officer husband Ian, in whom she quite rightly suspected I would have confided. He confirmed that I was in Kosovo, as did my sister Irene who lived near to Mum and was aware of my subterfuge. When I eventually took leave and visited Mum she asked me how I'd got on in America. Suspecting her motive, I came clean and apologized for the fib. I explained what I was involved in and told her that I'd be returning to Kosovo to continue the investigations. She told me she was really proud of my achievements, but mildly rebuked me for not telling her the truth in the beginning, although she understood that my decision not to do so was with her welfare in mind. The moral of this story? Never, ever tell fibs to your mum.

Chapter 31

The Village of Velika Kruša in Kosovo

Just when it looked like little or no further media attention would plague us, we learned that the FCO were sending the late Foreign Secretary Robin Cook on a goodwill visit. Their press people wanted him to join us at an exhumation site so that the British public could see us at work. We made arrangements to accommodate this request and a site at Velika Kruša was chosen. On the allotted day Mr Cook arrived in a flight of two military helicopters which landed close to the site in a field cleared and protected by NATO troops. At all of these sites those entering do so via a clean entrance and have to wear white paper suits, plastic overshoes, gloves and, where necessary, face masks in order not to contaminate the scene. The individual would exit via an unclean point where, after removing the protective clothing, which would be destroyed, they'd walk through a disinfected footbath and wash their hands and face in clean water. Mr Cook did this without fuss, but some of his entourage didn't want to wear protective clothing and were not too happy when told they therefore couldn't enter. One gent was so keen to remain with his boss that he got one leg in the suit, and then hopped behind him scrambling to complete his dress. Mr Cook had obviously done his homework. Questions he asked of the pathologist, anthros and police officers alike displayed a fair knowledge of our work. I personally knew one of his protection officers who confirmed this, adding that he (Cook) had read an FCO briefing note from top to bottom en route in the chopper.

Almost immediately the German Minister for Foreign Affairs, Herr Joschka Fischer, Robin Cook's equivalent arrived, again in a two-helicopter flight. These choppers were much heavier and the down draft they produced on landing caused some emergency tents set up near the field to accommodate refugee families to be blown away, their occupants and NATO soldiers scrambling after them with recovery in mind. The German minister went through the same disinfectant regime, but he spent much less time at the centre of the scene than Robin Cook. As he exited and began talking with a TV crew, one of his entourage had only just completed putting on a paper suit at the entry point. When he saw his boss had removed his at the exit point he promptly ripped his off, decided not to enter and instead joined his boss. What was the point, I thought? Had it not been for the serious nature of our work these antics would have been comical as well as ridiculous.

Chapter 32

Lapsed Security

Shortly after this it was time to escort some members of the BFT to Skopje Airport as their attachment had expired and to collect their replacements. Normally we did this using three of our off-road vehicles. On the mountainous route back in beautiful countryside very similar to that in Austria or Switzerland we passed through military roadblocks. We displayed UN stickers on the windscreens and rear windows of our vehicles, but otherwise they were unmarked. Often when we were about to drive through Serb villages the soldiers in the roadblocks would update us on the most recent security situation where necessary. We knew they would radio the next roadblock along the route reporting details of our convoy and our ETA at that roadblock.

At one US military roadblock we were simply waved through without any ID check or whatever, which was not unusual as our vehicles were pretty well known due to regular travel along this route. Approaching a particular Serb village we saw quite a large crowd in the marketplace so we slowed down assuming the crowd would let us pass, but there was no movement. A group of men approached our vehicles and started shouting and waving their arms about. Only the driver in the lead vehicle spoke the local language. He got out and began speaking with the main group leader so I alighted from my vehicle as did our ex-army explosives officer (expo) in the tail vehicle. Women in the group were yelling and ululating, which was not helping our plight.

It seemed that youths from the village had earlier that day been arrested by the US military and taken away. The villagers, especially relatives of these youths, fearing that their arrests were for war crimes were, to say the least, very upset. We explained our role in Kosovo and that we were unarmed UN forensic experts, but this was ignored. The group virtually encircled us and some of the newcomers to the BFT looked understandably confused and concerned. The noise level rose. The main man then told us we would be held hostage to be swapped for the arrested youths. He indicated we should slowly drive our cars into a nearby walled yard which normally held farm animals and park up, which we did. We all got out of our cars and reassured each other. Some had a ciggie, while others ate snacks they'd brought with them. With the expo and interpreter I spoke with the main man and asked to use our car radio to speak with the military. This was refused. I explained that the military in the roadblock further up the route would now be aware we were late so steps would be taken to check our progress. I offered to drive with him to this roadblock to find out what I could about the youths or to do so alone, then come back and tell him. These options were also declined.

After what seemed a very long time but in reality was no longer than just over an hour, we were extremely pleased and not a little relieved to see two Armoured Personnel Carriers (APCs) bearing Polish army insignia swing into the marketplace and about a dozen heavily-armed paratroopers alight and deploy around the crowd. An officer quickly ascertained that we were okay and told us to get into our cars and continue our journey. He also explained to the crowd that the youths had been arrested for disorder and stone-throwing at US troops and would be back in the village presently. This appeased the main man and his compatriots, but the women continued their screeching and wailing. They also annoyingly walked line abreast with linked arms across the roadway as slowly as they could for a good five minutes directly in front of our small convoy, no doubt ensuring that our journey would be delayed as a form of protest. I don't think I've ever been so glad to reach a roadblock. The troops here were also Polish (see photo plate section). They said we should have been warned about the arrests at the US roadblock and probably should have been escorted through by a military unit just in case the villagers took the sort of action they had. It seemed our European soldiers had more understanding of the Serb character than their American counterparts. Thankfully some of the new BFT members had arrived suitably armed with Johnnie Walker's finest, in which we made a dent at one of the safe houses later that eventful evening.

Chapter 33

Miscellany

On one of many occasions we were exhuming bodies from an embankment that required us to dig into the side of the bank instead of from above ground level as is normal, utilizing diggers from the local village who were mostly, if not all, relatives of the victims we were attempting to recover. As we took a short coffee break and the diggers shared their cigarettes (nearly every male smoked in this neck of the woods), we noticed a disturbance in the soil near these bodies. Suddenly a greasy, furry little head broke through with small paws frantically digging away the soil around it with two disgusting yellow rodent teeth prominent. The diggers went mad. They tried to kill it with their shovels, shouting loudly as they did so. The animal, which looked like a haggis with legs, ran between them but couldn't avoid the many spade strikes, so was soon killed. I learned it was a mole-rat which is exactly what it looked like: half mole, half rat. The locals detest them. Rumour has it that they eat cadavers. As they live underground and are virtually blind this may be the case. I must admit it was the ugliest rodent I've ever seen.

On the many and varied sites dealt with by the BFT, we worked alongside a number of different UK and NATO military units, many of whom were Territorial (part-time) soldiers and all of whom were extremely helpful and supportive to all our numerous requirements. Time and time again BFT staff were impressed with the professionalism and empathy of these squaddies. It was not unusual to see them organizing and participating in football and other games with children in these troubled villages. A team of British soldiers took on the task of repairing and rebuilding a village school that had been reduced to rubble by Serb artillery fire, most of which they did in their own time, no less. If my memory serves me well, we worked with and were protected by the Royal Regiment of Fusiliers (RRF), Royal Marines, Gurkha Regiment, Cheshire Regiment and Army Air Corps from the UK, while other NATO forces who assisted us whenever and wherever they could were from the USA, France, Germany, the Netherlands, Italy, Sweden, Finland, Russia, Poland and Norway.

During all this intensity and while I was back in the UK on R&R from BFT work I received a phone call from a Lab Sgt colleague which, for a change, was not a call to work; well, not my normal type of work, that is. My colleague had occasionally advised on TV programmes and the odd movie and had been approached by a film producer to do so on a film he was about to begin shooting in London. Alas, my pal would be abroad on leave and very kindly thought I could cover it. Why not? I could really do with an uplifting change from dealing with mass killings, even if it was only for a few days. After chatting to the producer, I attended the studio as required. The film was titled *Innocent Lies*, starring actors Adrian Dunbar as a detective and the ever-lovely Joanna Lumley as a murdered Mata Hari-type spy. The setting was Paris during the Great War. I advised on forensic techniques available to the police at that time and showed the actors portraying the cops how to take fingerprints and swabs, etc. At one stage in the film a detective sees an important piece of evidence lodged between the teeth of the victim, so for evidential purposes he removes it. I showed the actor how this would be done, but his hands were shaking as the camera rolled and several takes were attempted. The director asked me to carry out the procedure once more, which I did, not knowing that they continued to film. That footage, with my permission, was left in the movie so my hands appear in the film. It's a start, I suppose. Ironically I've never actually seen the film. I think, to use thespian slang, it 'bombed' in the cinemas. However, it was great fun to do and quite a pleasant change.

Chapter 34

Health & Safety

Summers in Kosovo can be pretty damn hot and when working a site out in the open we normally erected a couple of tents. One was a clean tent in which we stored water, snacks, consumable items and first-aid kits. Entry was restricted to personnel not contaminated or dirty. It was also a place to go for a bit of shade when it got too hot. The other was to store all the other stuff we carried and could be used to change clothes when it rained. A basic rule to which we tried to adhere was that when the temperature was hot, no-one should work for more than twenty minutes out in the open. Wearing paper suits made us sweat anyway, and digging and lifting heavy bodies quickly took its toll on some colleagues, even when hydrating regularly. I forgot this twenty-minute rule one day and became dizzy-headed and unwell. I told the crew I was going to lie down for a few minutes in the clean tent and strolled off to do so.

The next thing I knew someone was dabbing my face with a moist wipe and as I opened my eyes I realized I was lying between stacks of plastic water bottles and the person attending me was the lovely Julie Roberts, a fine anthro and former nurse. Looking over her shoulder and asking me if I was okay was one of the team pathologists. Be assured, you do not want to look into the eyes of a pathologist when you awaken, nice bloke though he was. Apparently I'd been fast asleep for quarter of an hour or so and they decided to check on me. Probably a combination of being overtired and spending too long out in the heat of the day. After hydrating sensibly I returned to my task and kept a strict eye on not only my own time in hot conditions but my colleagues' as well. In the spirit of true camaraderie, a while later they gifted me a photograph they'd taken of me in my slumbers. Thanks, guys…

I'd undertaken to replace the pathologist's field kit when the existing one became blunt and difficult to use given the many post-mortem examinations we were carrying out. This consisted of scalpels, knives, saws and probes required to carry out field autopsies contained within a black felt roll. I collected these from a Home Office facility in central London when on R&R, along with a letter of authority (LOA) signed by the Home Secretary. This permitted me to carry them on aircraft. On several trips I disclosed these items at the security check, produced the LOA and my police ID and was allowed to carry them on board in my rucksack.

However, on one occasion a security guard refused to let me board with them, demanding that they had to go in the hold. I told him they were too delicate for the hold and asked to speak with a supervisor. I explained the situation to him, informed him that I'd done this several times recently via this airport and airline and showed him the LOA. He stood by his colleague's decision, but offered a compromise. He ensured that it would be handed to the pilot and held in the cockpit during the flight. I could collect it from cabin crew at my destination. Under the circumstances I agreed, but reiterated that the instruments must be dealt with as very fragile. I boarded and was just settling down when a stewardess approached and asked me to confirm my ID. I showed her my police warrant card and UN ID plus the LOA. She handed me the instrument roll and told me they had no room in the cockpit so I'd have to look after it. With thanks, I promised to do so. No comment necessary...

It has been asked of me and many of my colleagues over the years just how we can do this line of work. That's hard to answer. I knew from very early on in my police career in Fife that death and the dying held no fear for me but rather I found investigating the same intriguing and fascinating, indeed a privilege. After all, there's no better task known to a detective than trying to establish the facts surrounding a person taking another person's life illegally, as the many professionals I've worked with over the years would concur. You're either able to switch off from the inhumanity of such occurrences and get on with your task or you are not. If the latter, you will not make the grade. This doesn't mean some cases don't get to you emotionally after the work is done. You'd be an automaton if this were the case. We've all shed a tear at some time or another.

During my first deployment in Kosovo in 1999 the FCO insisted that all team members underwent a counselling debriefing in a London hotel. I argued that for myself and a couple of the core members, who were all experienced detectives well accustomed to dealing with dead bodies, this was not necessary. I avoided saying that we were already beyond help because I knew this wouldn't go down well. They compromised, so we only had to attend one session when next returning to the UK for R&R. I felt they were a waste of time for me and I know a few other fellow professionals felt the same way. The counsellors, although undeniably well intentioned, had no experience of what we undertook on a daily basis. I suggested they should join us in situ and experience our daily lives, thus being better prepared to counsel other team members. I also put it on paper to the FCO who inferred that they would consider same. It never happened.

However, there was an occasion well into this period when my wife Sheila and I were on holiday on the beautiful Scottish Island of Skye when we were walking our dogs in the local mountain range known as the Cummins. While ascending a grassy knoll and looking around at the magnificent views I suddenly panicked, stopped in mid-step and stood absolutely stock still. For a moment I felt disorientated because I realized that I wasn't walking on a made and solid road. In other words I was standing in a potential minefield. On Skye? I shook myself and strode off. It never happened again, I'm happy to say. It was, of course, a stark reminder of the constant stress I'd been under for lengthy periods, as would be the case for many of my BFT colleagues.

Chapter 35

Political Murder in the Republic of Zambia

In November 1999 the government of the Republic of Zambia requested that the FCO supply a Scotland Yard CID team to undertake an independent investigation into the recent murder of a leading opposition politician. I was still writing up reports and giving presentations concerning BFT work in Kosovo as well as regularly responding to suspicious deaths almost on a daily basis. Regardless of this, I was still 'in the barrel' which means on the FCO call-out list for such international demands. It didn't surprise me therefore when a highly-respected and competent MIT Det Supt, Steve Gwilliam, with whom I'd worked on several murders, called me to join him as his forensic adviser for an investigation into a politically sensitive murder in Zambia. Guess what my response was? With his DI Peter we flew to Lusaka the following day where a couple of senior uniform police officers met us, ushered us to a pair of sparkling new stretch Mercedes cars and drove us to their police HQ. As we drove along my eyes were drawn to a gilded Kalashnikov AK-47 automatic rifle clipped to the dashboard. Different…

Our hosts briefed us about the murder of a United National Independence Party (UNIP) candidate for Lusaka who was the son of former President Kenneth Kaunda, namely Major Wezi Kaunda, fatally shot outside his address in Kabulonga district as he and his wife arrived home from a political function. According to his wife Didri, at least four armed men approached their vehicle as he alighted to open their garage gate. He told them who he was and told them to take the vehicle and not harm anyone. According to Didri one of the men said they knew who he was, then one of them shot him in the stomach. She was ordered out of the car while the men piled in and drove it off. Police later found it abandoned nearby. Nothing had been taken from it. Armed car hijacking is a regular and prominent crime in Zambia.

There was a slight delay in our being allowed to start our enquiry which would take diplomatic handling according to a representative of the British Embassy who suggested we fill the time by meeting the father of the deceased in order to obtain a better understanding of the political situation in the country, so the three of us attended ex-President Kaunda's impressive home where we were led by liveried staff to a large acacia tree in the garden to await our host. A bench ran around this tree which offered thankful shade. A short while later the ex-president emerged. He was a formidable presence carrying his ever-present fly whisk and dressed in a smart, dark blue safari suit in which I'd often seen him in photographs holding a similar fly whisk seated beside HM The Queen at Commonwealth ministers meetings.

He exchanged a few pleasantries with us and asked one of his staff to fetch refreshments. Steve introduced himself and Peter and as he introduced me as the forensic input on the team Mr Kaunda asked me a few questions on the subject. As I replied, he said: 'You're not English, are you?' I told him I was proud to be a Scot from the Kingdom of Fife. He smiled and told me that his father had been a missionary and teacher ordained in the Church of Scotland and that one of his daughters obtained her degree at St Andrews University in Fife. As our refreshments arrived he jokingly asked if I'd prefer anything stronger, hinting that he enjoyed a drop of whisky himself. I think Steve was wondering what was going on at this stage. Normal service was resumed. We later met the ex-president's daughter and as she spoke I noted that she still had a slight Scottish burr. The ex-president was of the opinion that as his son Wezi had been a severe threat to the governing political party he had been the subject of a political assassination disguised to look like a car hijacking carried out by common criminals.

When we got the go-ahead I met two Zambian police CID officers who'd been trained in forensic recovery. They showed me their office in the police HQ building which was in a very dilapidated state. Many windows were broken or hanging from their frames, doors were missing or hanging off the hinges and car wrecks filled the yard. They were proud to show me their two Zeiss crime scene cameras that were gifted to them when the Brits left during Zambia's independence in the 1960s. Unbelievably, the film for these was held by the duty Supt to whom they had to apply as and when they needed to use the cameras. They had next to no evidence packaging and no transport, but were remarkably keen and able.

We all visited the scene of the crime and discussed how to conduct further enquiries, after which I took a detailed look at the deceased's vehicle, a Toyota GX Land Cruiser, in the police yard. From this examination I roughly determined the position of the gunman and from talking with the deceased's widow Didri estimated where her husband stood when he was shot. A return to the scene resulted in the recovery of two 7.62mm bullet heads in soil. This is the calibre of bullet fired from Kalashnikov AK-47 automatic rifles. Unfortunately they are ten a penny in this continent, but if police recovered the actual weapon used we could compare them to confirm usage.

A senior Zambian police officer informed us that they'd identified the gang responsible and hoped to arrest them soon. The gang leader was known to be extremely dangerous; in fact too dangerous for us to be present during his arrest, he insisted. Steve suggested that we held briefings with all of the officers assigned to this investigation in the manner of Scotland Yard. This was agreed in principle but the inspectors demanded a separate briefing and the NCOs preferred to be separated from the constables. It wasn't going to work. We'd already noted that subordinate ranks didn't speak up when a senior officer was present. The other problem was that although they all carried Kalashnikov AK-47 rifles, none of them possessed a notebook or writing material.

Another suggestion was to set up a roadblock at the murder scene around the time it had happened with a view to obtaining any passing witnesses that had not yet come forward. This was approved, so we set up information boards and emergency lighting as it would be dusk, and briefed uniform officers who would be wearing high-visibility clothing to man the roadblock and stop and speak with drivers. We'd be present throughout. A traffic car and motorcycle were to stand by in case anyone refused to stop.

More or less the first car that approached slowed down, swerved off the road around the officers and accelerated away. I jumped into the traffic car and we gave chase, stopping it a few minutes later. I approached the driver who was a lone European female and showed her my ID. She opened her window ever so slightly, then ranted at me for frightening her. She went on to say no lone female would stop for such a roadblock, fearing that they were not real police. Zambian police never did this, she said. She was the spouse of a foreign diplomat who, like many others, travelled that route around the same time each evening. I apologized for our naïvety and distress caused, then handed her my card containing our local telephone number and asked if she would speak to any other users of the route to see if they had witnessed anything. We then escorted her to her compound nearby. It was decided to abort the roadblock fiasco, although I still think it was worth trying.

Zambian police officers carried out a number of raids whereby four of the suspected gang members were now in custody. A fifth man, the alleged extremely dangerous leader, had resisted arrest and was fatally shot by police. All were brought to police HQ. Over the next few days we assisted with ID parades during which Didri, after several attempts, picked out two of the men. This would have been unacceptable in a UK case. A bizarre form of ID parade comprising dead bodies and the shot gang leader's corpse was held in a local mortuary, again asking Didri to see if she could identify any suspect. This was unsuccessful, even given that the suspect's body was literally riddled with bullets unlike the other cadavers that had died of natural causes or in road accidents, of which there are many in the roads around Lusaka. The latter ID was the brainchild of Zambian police. We took no part; in fact Steve had strongly advised against it. All four men arrested were charged with the murder of Major Wezi Kaunda and other related serious crimes, then lengthy court proceedings began.

I brought the fact that the Zambian police forensic unit had little or no equipment to the attention of the Department for International Development (DFID), as well as the fact that I'd been made aware that the Met had about ten former SOCO mini-vans which were due to be scrapped. At minimal cost, some of these could be salvaged and repaired, painted in Zambian police livery and fitted out for forensic use, then shipped out to Zambia for police use. Both forensic officers we'd met and worked with would be offered advanced forensic training at Hendon. A win/win situation for them, I'm sure.

Chapter 36

The BFT and I Return to Kosovo: 2000

The BFT and I returned to Kosovo in 2000, would you believe the day before my 52nd birthday, with yours truly in the same role as in 1999 to continue this vitally important work. Again financed by the FCO, we were tasked to carry out another lengthy mission to recover hundreds of bodies and a great deal of evidence for future use within trials at the ICTY in The Hague. Because the Met had provided most of the police officers, photographers and SOCOs for the 1999 mission, staff for this mission were drawn from other English police forces and the much-revered Royal Ulster Constabulary (RUC) of Northern Ireland. The lead SIO was DCS Steve Watts, Head of Hampshire Constabulary CID, an experienced and dedicated detective with a good track record.

I first met Steve when he and I were invited to a meeting within the FCO chaired by Catherine Nettleton, CMG, OBE, at that time the War Crimes Co-ordinator for the former Yugoslavia. It would be fair to say that he was not all that enamoured with having me, a Met DS who he did not know from Adam nor had he any idea about my level of competence, foisted upon him as the BFT coordinator but Ms Nettleton kindly insisted, citing my unrivalled experience in this post. Understandably Steve had an experienced Hants colleague in mind for the role. It didn't take long, however, once we started working together in theatre, for a mutual understanding and trust to be formed. At the conclusion of the 2000 mission Steve wrote a flattering and humbling letter to my ultimate boss at Scotland Yard, Assistant Commissioner Crime (ACC) Dave Veness, CBE, QPM, not only praising my professionalism during the tour but additionally recommending me for a Commissioner's Commendation. I proudly received same in the presence of my wife and daughters shortly thereafter from Metropolitan Police Commissioner John Stevens, QPM, KStJ himself.

Along with another core member William 'Billy' Fulton, who was a DS in the RUC with considerable anti-terrorism experience obtained during 'the Troubles' in Northern Ireland and who had been part of the 1999 BFT, I was despatched to the Kosovan capital of Pristina to link up with the various agencies with whom we would be working as well as to reconnoitre suitable safe accommodation. We initially rented rooms in the truly awful UN Hotel within the UN compound, where a couple of nights later we were disturbed by an explosion then resultant fire in a nearby house. By virtue of his experience in Northern Ireland, Billy recognized that it had been caused by a type of rifle-launched rocket. A few UN civilian staff in rooms on our floor were rather upset and concerned that more rockets may follow as we heard the sirens of approaching fire and police units. We suggested that they bring a chair out on to the hallway where there was some shelter and no windows and when that was done we shared a bottle of Scottish or maybe Irish single malt with those who imbibed to keep them calm.

It became increasingly difficult to determine who the BFT could work with as senior UN police and ICTY personnel told us that the UN per se would not authorize them to liaise with the BFT at that time. These colleagues were well aware of our work capability and achievements the year before and would welcome any opportunity to work with us again; however, historically slow and cumbersome UN administration prevented that from happening. The paperwork, which the FCO insisted was in order, was most definitely not. Even staff at the British Consulate, although sympathetic, could not assist with our plight. A compromise was to have Ms Nettleton attend so that she could sign anew the required Memoranda of Understanding (MOU) with the various parties, thus permitting us to start work. This the good lady did, allowing us to kick-start bringing the team in. Steve joined us soon thereafter and following a number of further meetings with those in charge of the UN departments, civil authority and military leaders, agreements were reached for the BFT to more or less pick up from where we had left off in 1999.

House-hunting had progressed quite well. Billy and I had identified a couple of potential properties that could accommodate the entire team securely and in a safe and reasonably accessible area. We left the fiscal side to Consular staff while we got on with arrangements to utilize the mortuary facilities in Pristina Hospital. The previous year's BFT vehicles were delivered to us from the British Embassy in Skopje, Macedonia.

Equipment, protective clothing and consumables were ordered and would be flown in from RAF Brize Norton, West Oxfordshire in the UK to Skopje along with the initial team.

Again sites were identified by ICTY investigators on the ground in keeping with the requirements of tribunal prosecutors at The Hague who were poring over evidence retrieved from many sources. Any evidence retrieved would again be used in the upcoming trials of war criminals. I was to spend more than six months on this mission, made new friends and contacts, and met up with experts with whom I'd worked before. As the initial team flew in I looked forward to again linking up with a colleague and friend Michael Clarke (aka 'Swampy' because of his desire to get involved; in fact get into every grave site, no matter how unpleasant), a West Yorkshire police officer who was renowned for his empathy and rapport with the relatives of the deceased who attended the sites. He was a highly-rated team member for whom nothing was too much trouble; loved and respected by all. Swampy is also the cheeriest bloke I know, who kept our spirits up on many occasions.

Mention of the 2000 Kosovo tour could not be complete without the highest of praise for our military colleagues in the NATO-led Kosovo International Peacekeeping Force (KFOR). This incorporated primarily a Norwegian army engineer battalion that undertook nearly all the heavy-duty exhumations. They also provided us with body recovery and explosives search dogs when necessary as well as excellent 'Norge' hospitality on more than one occasion. The respect within the BFT for this military unit was immense. They truly lived up to their motto 'Nothing is Impossible' time after time. They were held in such high esteem by us that when the BFT polo shirt badge was designed, it incorporated the Norwegian flag beneath the Union Jack (see photo plate section).

We were also very well looked after by the RUC contingent of some sixty-five men and women who policed the Pristina area under the UN banner keeping the peace in a war zone, which is never easy and not without danger. They simultaneously trained local police recruits in more acceptable and less segregationist policing methods. Their professional assistance and liaison role on behalf of the police officers attached to our mission should not be underestimated. Their continued support and security advice throughout our deployment reassured us. No doubt Pristina was a much safer place because of their presence on the streets and in the neighbouring villages, many of which were potential flash-points for continued ethnic violence and civil disturbances.

For a lengthy period we operated in Dragonara Cemetery situated just outside Pristina. Here a number of murdered victims had been buried between legal graves mainly dug by Romany gypsies who affiliated themselves with the Serbian military during the war. The equivalent of a cemetery superintendent had been located and with the aid of his records we were able to distinguish the legal from illegal burials. We slowly progressed with this grisly task, always under KFOR protection by the Royal Regiment of Fusiliers (RRF), readily identifiable by the distinctive white and red plume on their berets, a battle honour from Napoleonic days. These soldiers, like many others, selflessly manned our outer and, where it was more hazardous, the inner security cordons to enable the BFT to work on in safety and without unauthorized interruption.

The majority of these squaddies were quite young and many were interested in what we were doing. When the situation allowed we'd let them have a closer look at our findings and sometimes the anthro and pathology work at field post-mortem examinations, with the proviso that no photos be taken. Several days into this dig a captain from the regiment, accompanied by their padre, paid us a visit. It seemed they were concerned that a few of their soldiers were finding our work distressing so asked not to be assigned to inner cordon duties. I was perplexed. The officers explained that very few of their soldiers had ever seen a dead person up close and the few that had had only seen relatives who'd died of natural causes. The majority had only viewed dead bodies in film clippings of war casualties during basic training. It was agreed to limit his soldiers' close attendance forthwith. We had a very good working relationship with them throughout this aspect of the mission. As most of the BFT crew had regular involvement with violent death, post mortems and the like, it hadn't occurred to us that soldiers would find the nature of our work upsetting. Another lesson learned.

There were times when I was personally torn between going home to my wife and family as the stresses and consistent pressure mounted. I was seeing, in fact experiencing first-hand, the misery and desperation on the faces of relatives of these many, many victims on a daily basis, and had been doing so for several years now. I would regularly sit with relatives of the missing, presumed dead, in each village on our list to discuss how we were to conduct the extraction of their lost and loved ones when I'd realize that their need and expectations far exceeded my personal feelings. Onwards and upwards it was then.

My younger daughter Ceri was in the middle of a gap year from university at this time and was travelling around Australia with several girlfriends. She'd kept in regular touch with her mother and me; however, after sending a postcard to her mum stating where she was heading next, she'd not been in touch for a while. Her mum discovered a frightening news item that there had been a fatal fire in a backpackers' youth hostel near the town of Childers in Queensland, where Ceri was allegedly headed, so she got in touch with me somewhat distressed to see what I could find out. To say the least I could do very little from Kosovo so initially I sent texts and left messages on Ceri's phone requesting her to contact me pronto. No response. Understandably her mum was in a state. I wasn't much better to be honest. I contacted senior colleagues at New Scotland Yard explaining my concern and was gratified in the knowledge that they were able to liaise with the Australian Federal Police dealing with this fatal fire. All they could ascertain at this early stage of the investigation, however, was that no-one with our daughter's surname was booked into the hostel. It was a little reassuring and gave us hope that she was simply out of phone range, hopefully enjoying her travels, safe and sound... Please God. I was not in the habit of praying, not being a particular believer in any God given what I'd experienced in my professional life, but I confess I did ask for any supreme being's assistance to ensure her safety.

Sure enough, a short time later I received a phone call from Ceri in which she outlined her recent travels and wondered what all the fuss was about. I explained our concerns and told her to contact her mum straight away, then call me back when she'd done so. It transpired she'd been on a three-day sailing course with her friends, living on board while out at sea where their phones didn't work. They had not reached Childers. The elation and relief I felt were overwhelming and I must be honest I did shed a tear, as did a female BFT colleague who knew my dilemma and who was with me at breakfast in an army camp when I received Ceri's call. Although my loved one was alive and well, I soon realized how awful it must have been for the many relatives we'd encountered to not know what had happened to their loved ones and the feeling of helplessness this brings. Having said that, I also felt pangs of guilt too. Fifteen backpackers had died in the inferno, which local investigators would prove to be an act of deliberate arson, so while I was mentally celebrating our good luck, the relatives of these fifteen unfortunate youngsters were going through their own type of hell. An itinerant Aussie drifter responsible for this arson deservedly received a sentence of life imprisonment. I was also extremely grateful to the Scotland Yard and Australian Federal Police officers who'd shared some of their data with me. Surely camaraderie of the finest order.

The female colleague who shed a tear with me when I learned that Ceri was safe and sound was herself a DS in the RUC who went on to take charge of that force's DVI (Disaster Victim Identification) unit and accomplish numerous body recoveries at the tragic 2004 Indian Ocean tsunami. A former nurse and a fine lass, she did, however, have a bit of difficulty remembering the names of the various tools used during grave exhumations: items such as trowels, mattocks and scalpels. When she was working in a grave it was not uncommon for her to request (in her lilting Northern Irish brogue), 'Could somebody please pass me the thingy?' When an unsuitable tool was passed to her she'd regale her colleague with: 'Not that thingy, I need the wee thingy.' To this day I get the occasional text from her signed off 'Thingy'. By the way, if you ever watch *Time Team* or similar archaeological dig programmes you'll notice that the more experienced an archaeologist is, the smaller their trowel. This denotes their experience as the metal diminishes after a lot of usage. Some wear it like a badge of office, but most simply get on with the fine work at hand.

It is fair to say that each discipline within the BFT complemented the others and no single unit could have completed the volume and quality of work without the other. However, in my now quite informed opinion, forensic anthropologists were irreplaceable when it came to a complete recovery of grave contents. It is my firm belief as a result that no exhumation should be carried out without one of these experts present, whether it be a single victim of domestic murder or a mass co-mingled war grave (see photo plate section).

197

By the end of the 2000 assignment the BFT had examined 46 sites, recovering 445 bodies consisting of 307 males, 93 females and 45 unknown because of skeletal disruption; 209 were identified. Other international exhumation teams over the same period examined 237 sites and recovered 1,390 bodies consisting of 955 males, 195 females and 240 unknown; 997 were identified. Overall during this two-year period international exhumation teams, including the BFT, examined 429 sites and recovered 3,620 bodies consisting of 2,798 males, 481 females and 341 unknown; 2,099 were identified. Quite an achievement, for sure.

Steve, Billy, Clarkie and myself, as BFT core members, were subsequently awarded the UN Kosovo campaign medal because of our longevity in that theatre of war and no doubt the excellent results that all in the BFT had attained. We accepted this honour with pride on behalf of all of the marvellous BFT personnel.

Shortly before I retired from the Met the Press Bureau at Scotland Yard were obviously looking for a good PR story so they asked if I'd agree to journalist Robert Chesshyre, who had previously written a newspaper article on JG, spending some time with me in my capacity as a Lab Sgt in order to feature me in a newspaper article to include my taking up my new role with the ICTY. I was naturally flattered, so after checking with JG that I could rely on Bob's discretion I accepted.

I called Bob out to several murder and suspicious death crime scenes and resultant post mortems over the next few weeks to give him a flavour of the work conducted by the LLOs on a daily basis. I needn't have been concerned about Bob's discretion as I found him to be a consummate professional and we soon became good chums, trusting one another. I still on occasions meet up with him and JG for a spot of lunch in central London.

His article was published in the *Sunday Telegraph* magazine on 9 March 2002 under the heading 'Burden of Proof' where he detailed our experiences over his weeks as a 'fly on the wall' journalist. I was pleased with it, apart from where in his description of me he used the word 'bulky', even though he was correct. Obviously he meant to type 'well-built'. More importantly, my mum was really, really chuffed. At the end of the article Bob wrote a few lines that I think are particularly pertinent to the work I'd already been involved in and the work I was about to take on with the ICTY. These were [Turnbull's mission at The

Hague is] 'to create an evidence trail that will lead from the blood-stained ravines of the Balkans to the dock.' How right he was, and how proud I was to have been able to play a part in the various organizations that accomplished this.

Chapter 37

The Start of Another Career in the United Nations

'The United Nations was not created to take mankind to heaven, but to save humanity from hell.'

Dag Hammarskjöld
Second UN Secretary-General, 1954

Having been actively involved in war crime investigations in the Balkans since 1996, seconded as described to the UN via the FCO, I was offered a post by UN ICTY at The Hague in 2002 which I proudly accepted. This required my retirement from the Met after thirty-five years' service which was acclaimed on the Certificate of Service I received from the commissioner's office as 'Exemplary'. I took charge of the ICTY Evidence Unit which not only dealt with the evidence against notorious Serbian politicians Slobodan Milošević and Radovan Karadžić but Serb military leader General Ratko Mladić who was in charge of overrunning the UN Dutch Battalion's designated safe zone near Srebrenica, causing the massacre of an almost unbelievable total in excess of 8,000 Muslim men and boys. The unit also provided vital evidence in the lengthy trials of all the other major war criminals indicted from the former Yugoslavia to face charges of war crimes, ethnic cleansing and other human rights atrocities.

My function there was to ensure that the integrity of this hard-won evidence was maintained and that it be available for analysis and research by the investigators and attorneys tasked with bringing these cases to court at the tribunal. Initially I had around forty excellent staff who were responsible for more than 3.8 million evidential documents, a great many of which were electronic intercepts of military and police conversations, and in excess of 6,000 hours of video evidence, over and above large quantities of physical artefacts. We constantly reviewed potential new methods of electronic stamping/scanning/editing of these items and as a result modified to a fully digitized system to protect the video evidence from degrading, some of which had originally come to the unit in poor condition some seven or eight years earlier.

My good friends ex-DS Cliff Smith from the Met and ex-DS Billy Fulton of the RUC had likewise joined the ranks of the ICTY as investigators, so I had them to fall back on if I came across any hiccups in the organization. Both were still actively engaged in detailed enquiries back in Kosovo, but from time to time returned to The Hague which was also good on the social side of life. I was living in a fine rented apartment overlooking the beautiful park in front of The Hague Central Rail Station. My landlord Peter, who lived on the floor above, was a retired Dutch diplomat with whom I spent pleasant and informative hours chatting over coffee and tasty home-made biscuits prepared by his charming Macedonian wife Wilma. During the Nazi occupation of the Netherlands in the Second World War the block was requisitioned as quarters for Gestapo officers. The European Police Organization (Europol) building nearby was similarly acquired as the Gestapo interrogation and detention HQ. On entering my block a large sweeping stairway led up three floors. On the plinths at each side of the banister at ground-floor level sat two impressive bronze eagles. In my mind's eye I could envisage a red-collared senior Gestapo officer escorting a lady of the night up this stairway to his chambers for an evening of distraction from the war. My landlord was a member of an organization attempting to retrieve paintings and other works of art stolen by the Nazis from their Dutch and mainly Jewish owners during this occupation.

Members of the Evidence Unit continued to attend locations in the Balkans, even at this late stage, to assist with recovery of evidence. I visited the sister UN tribunal in Tanzania, tasked with investigating the atrocities in Rwanda, in order to confer with my counterpart there with the intention of setting up similar effective evidence pipelines that they were using very successfully and generally learn from one another's experiences.

As ICTY attorneys prepared indictments against these war criminals, the Evidence Unit updated them as to what corroborative evidence was held in the vaults pertinent to each case. In order to preserve the integrity of these items, or even worse in case of the loss of any of them, they were scanned where possible and the scan secured for court purposes. The ICTY possessed an internal CCTV system so an attorney in court could call up the scanned exhibits for all to view and discuss without having to draw the original item out of the vault. This worked very well.

Occasionally with other specialists I'd travel to various locations in Kosovo as part of a training team to pass on our experience of war crime investigation to magistrates, lawyers, police officers and anyone else involved with bringing the lower-level war criminals, if there are such beings, before local courts. Although most participants seemed keen, it was to take much longer than anticipated to get this process off the ground.

In 2003 my good friend Cliff sadly succumbed to Gaucher's disease after courageously fighting it for quite some time. This pervasive genetic disorder can cause an enlarged spleen and liver malfunction, as well as a very painful skeletal disorder. Cliff collapsed while carrying out ICTY investigations in Kosovo and was diagnosed as suffering from this ailment after the UN flew him over to a hospital in Leiden, the Netherlands.

One of the most difficult things I've ever had to do was present a eulogy at the celebration of his life held in Leiden in the presence of his wife Angela and their four lovely young children who I obviously knew very well. Angela chose to remain in the Netherlands, where I had the privilege of seeing all the Smith clan progress through life, graduate from university and each secure a good career. The work ethic of both Cliff and Angela shone through. RIP buddy.

Chapter 38

All Work and No Play

All work and no play makes Jack a dull boy as the saying goes, which makes a great deal of sense to me and those of us engaged in what at times can be frustrating, depressing, gruesome and hazardous work. It is important for morale and the wellbeing of personnel for those with the responsibility of management to ensure that a bit of more light-hearted activity is built into their lives when engaged far from home in conditions that are far from perfect and with people they may not have known or worked with before.

The BFT spent a fair amount of time during 2000 working with and under the protection of an engineering unit of the Norwegian army, most of whom, male and female, were part-time soldiers. They were exceedingly professional and when we could we socialized together. The entire BFT team was invited to join them at their barracks one afternoon to watch a televised soccer match featuring Norway in an international competition. Their barracks, which I'd visited often for lunch and meetings with their mine-clearing teams and dog-handlers over the months, had been a JNA (former Yugoslav army) barracks which NATO had bombed and which the Norge reconstructed for their own use. As we prepared transport, a couple of female members of the BFT, an anthro and a SOCO, told me they were not interested in football and might stay behind and rest. I thought it would be good if we all attended and talked them into coming along.

An extensive marquee was set up with a large screen on which the football match would be viewed and there was a liberal bar. Many of our hosts had their national flag painted on their faces and wore their nation's football kit. There was almost a carnival feeling in the air. Throughout the region when we first arrived in theatre the place was scattered with broken-down and sometimes shot-up Zastava motor cars. These were the Serbian equivalent of the small Fiat 600 cars very popular all over Europe in the 1960s through to the 80s. The Norge had collected a few of these left abandoned, cut off the roofs, repaired the engines and painted them in their national colours. The result was a fleet of sort of golf buggies which soldiers drove around the large barracks area. As we awaited the start of the football game, I noticed our two somewhat reluctant ladies at the bar surrounded by a group of young, fit Norge squaddies so I ambled over and asked if they were alright. With a cheeky grin, the anthro smiled and mouthed words to the effect that they 'were fine, thanks'. I left them to it.

As the opening music roared ever more loudly from the many stereo loudspeakers throughout the marquee, the unmistakeable rumble of a heavy Leopard assault tank, of which our hosts had several, came ever nearer. Suddenly a tent flap was drawn open and the CO of the regiment stood saluting as he was driven into the arena in one of these small Zastava cars bearing a large loudspeaker emitting the sound of the tank. We all applauded this fine prank, after which the CO welcomed the guests and invited all to have an enjoyable evening. When the game started we all became Norge supporters, obviously. These social events offered us brief shafts of joyous sunlight in the otherwise grey pallor of our far from normal and often grim days.

At another location our protection force and mechanical excavator operators were from the Gurkha regiment. I've never seen such hard-working individuals in my life. Again the BFT was invited to a mess night with them where we partook of the finest goat curry most of us had ever enjoyed. As a proud Scot it was also great to hear the bagpipers. Speaking of same, I was a privileged guest as a representative of the BFT of the Head of the British Office in Pristina, Mr David Slinn, to HM The Queen's official birthday celebrations that year. I stood on the podium with him and Brigadier Richard Shirreff, CO of the British Forces Kosovo and several COs from other British KFOR regiments who I'd met before. One of them, who'd probably detected my Scots accent, as a flute and drum band marched by asked me if I enjoyed military bands and when I responded positively, adding that it's always much better with some bagpipes, he told me he thought I'd be of that opinion. At this the band were carrying out an 'about turn' move and from behind a container they were joined by four pipers. The officer smiled, as did I, then he added: 'I'm given to understand The Queen enjoys them too.'

While operating with the world-famous Royal Marines (RM), I carried out a forward recce to locate an alleged mass grave in the hills of Kosovo with two Commandos as mine-clearance experts, and two paramedics in case of any mishap accompanied by their padre who wanted to see how his troops worked with the BFT. Or perhaps he just wanted to get out of the camp for a while? After several hours mapping out the site in the summer heat, we were all pretty dusty and thirsty, and we drove past a large lake that was too good to miss. Ensuring that no-one was in the vicinity – it was a remote area, after all – we went in for a refreshing swim. I don't think any of my friends or colleagues have ever 'skinny-dipped' with four Commando NCOs and their officer, a man of the cloth for goodness sake, in a war zone. By the way, the RM padre had earned the much-revered green beret of the RM Commando in the same way as all others by passing their most gruelling fitness programme. The only difference was that during his field training he didn't fire a weapon; however, he had to carry the same weight as his combatant colleagues. The NCO during his final test ensured that this was a heavy machine gun.

RM paramedics are also bandsmen and women who wear a blue naval beret, not the distinctive green of the Commandos. They invited the BFT to an evening of music where they performed their version of *The Blues Brothers* movie. We were requested to arrive at their barracks at a specific time and in so doing were kept outside the hangar by a medic we knew well for a brief period. At a prearranged musical note (we later found out), we were led in at that point in the film when the Blues Brothers on stage welcome the law enforcement officers pursuing them into the stadium. In this case the BFT were the law enforcement agency stand-ins. The music was brilliant, as was their hospitality. They really are a unique regiment.

Also during 2000 Fulton and I were conducting a forward recce in a Finnish army protection zone in a highland region of Kosovo. Making our way back to the Finnish camp, I was driving a BFT Land Rover Discovery while Billy took a nap. In fairness, it had been a gruelling hot day. I was following a half-tracked coupled vehicle down a steep, scree-ridden slope between trees and at times had very little forward vision because of the dust and scree kicked up by this vehicle. I became aware, too late, that I'd run out of track. I should have veered left after the Finnish vehicle, but unfortunately had gone straight on. Realizing my error, I swerved too sharply to the left. The 'Disco' didn't like it, so we rolled, only once thank goodness, but enough to awaken Billy.

A group of saplings about 4 or 5 metres further down the mountainside fortunately stopped our descent. A bit shaken, slightly bruised and very embarrassed, I heard our escort shouting for us not to move. No problem; we weren't going anywhere. It took a while to winch us up, then we took it a bit slower while effecting our descent.

As it was becoming dark, it was decided we should remain in the Finnish army camp. Road travel back to Pristina was hazardous at the best of times, but in the dark it would have been downright dangerous. The Finnish major arranged overnight accommodation for us, then cordially invited us for a sauna which sounded like a great idea. The Finns don't bother with towels like we prudish Brits. Once inside, we Brits of course sat cross-legged while chatting and enjoying the cleansing, relaxing heat. The major banged on the wall, which we later learned was an adjoining sauna for NCOs, and then a naked soldier came in. Drinks were duly ordered, delivered and enjoyed, then our host said he normally ended a sauna session with a dip in the pool. Still 'sans towels', we walked a few metres to a shallow pool which they'd built specially and dipped straight in. Apart from wanting to cool down, the presence of female soldiers walking about nearby quickened our step and lessened our embarrassment. We shared a really good meal and the privileges of the Finnish military mess bar before sleeping like babies. After a rousing brekkie, we headed for Pristina with a greater appreciation of our other Scandinavian hosts.

Readers may recall I mentioned earlier (see Chapter 8) that before I joined the Met I'd written to the RCMP offering my services, but never received a reply. Just before I became embroiled in all the UN mass grave work in the Balkans I found myself, in the capacity of Homicide Advisor, on a non-stop overnight flight from London Heathrow to Vancouver, Canada to link up with a Vancouver Metropolitan Police homicide expert and a lovely lady biologist colleague from MPFSL who specialized in the study of rape and sexual deviant behaviour. Our joint task was to provide fresh eyes and minds reviewing a number of as yet unsolved sexually motivated homicides in that region, as well as a lengthy ongoing serial murder enquiry being carried out by law enforcement agencies in Seattle, USA. The media had labelled this latter series of homicides the Green River Murders due to the fact that the first five of the many female victims' bodies linked to this killer were discovered in the vicinity of that river between the 1980s and 90s. We discussed in detail these crime scenes with the investigators and read reports covering such homicides over many years.

During these reviews I was coerced into giving a presentation to a criminology class at the Simon Fraser University, Vancouver and later met a deputy commissioner from the RCMP. Over coffee during a general chit-chat I mentioned that I'd written to his force many years before applying for a post but had never received a reply. He kindly asked if I wanted him to chase it up; pretty much tongue in cheek, of course. We agreed with a chuckle that given I was only a couple of years away from completing thirty years' police service and therefore then able to retire, I was unlikely to be offered a transfer. Nice thought though: me, a Mountie!

Part of my brief for this mission was also to evaluate the RCMP evidence retrieval system and how Canadian law enforcement agencies recorded and disseminated forensic intelligence gleaned from major crime investigations using a system known as VICLAS (Violent Crime Linkage Analysis System), similar to the one generated by the FBI and known as VICAP (Violent Criminal Apprehension Program) in the US. I was tasked to compare these systems against how we carried out this function in the UK where police forces compiled a Criminal Record Office (CRO) Form 74 which contained identity details of the perpetrator, the modus operandi (method of operation of the crime) and generated a unique reference that stayed with the suspect if convicted.

VICLAS was designed to track and correlate information on violent crime, especially murder. RCMP provided the software for the database which is widely used by state and local law enforcement agencies to compile information on the following:

- sexual assault cases
- solved and unsolved homicides, especially those involving a kidnapping or if they are apparently motiveless, sexual or random or suspected to be part of a series
- missing persons, where foul play is suspected
- unidentified persons, where foul play is suspected.

To help me with this I was permitted to ride along with an RCMP equivalent of a SOCO for a couple of days while he responded to major crime scene calls. It just so happened that he'd been a former Met CID officer who'd transferred to the RCMP a few years beforehand and was now one of their Crime Scene Investigators. It was obvious that the way in which he dealt with crime scene work was virtually a mirror of how we did things in the Met. He'd found it relatively straightforward when he transferred, he told me.

I was surprised to learn that the RCMP had a particular problem with biker crime, which we didn't have in the UK, so much of their VICLAS data reflected the drive-by shootings, murders, interstate drug-smuggling and bombings between rival gangs of the Hell's Angel variety; much more violent than in the UK. Accordingly a large portion of VICLAS paperwork was not relevant to the British police. CRO74s only needed a bit of tweaking in my opinion, as I declared in my advisory report to Scotland Yard upon my return.

For the record in 2001 Gary Leon Ridgway was arrested in Washington State as the 'Green River Killer'. He eventually admitted to seventy-one murders in the Green River Killer portfolio and due to plea bargaining in which he disclosed the locations of a number of his still missing victims, he avoided the death sentence. He was convicted of forty-nine homicides and sentenced to life imprisonment without parole. His victims were raped and then strangled, initially manually but later on via ligature. He admitted often returning to the shallow graves and committing necrophilia on many of these unfortunate women. Law enforcement agencies believe that the real total of his murdered victims is nearer ninety, most of whom, certainly initially, were sex workers, runaways and vulnerable females. He is considered to be America's most prolific serial killer.

Chapter 39

Beware of Mines

A constant awareness of land mines and booby traps was required throughout these deployments and as each new member joined, they were given a presentation on this most important subject. Paramount to all of our safety, it was emphasized that especially in larger grave sites where cordons were placed that we kept an eye on one another lest someone should wander off into an uncleared area. This was particularly relevant when no toilet facilities were available and staff had to utilize the cover of trees and other vegetation to relieve themselves. As more female staff joined the BFT, we were required to provide on-site portable loos. Blokes had been happy enough previously au naturel. An RAF medic sent a request to the German military camp responsible for the region we'd be working in next, providing a grid reference as to where we needed the Portaloo delivered the following day. As we set up camp we saw a German army truck drive past and place a bright blue Portaloo in a nearby field. As the truck returned our RAF buddy hailed it and explained that it was ours and should be here. In true Teutonic form, he was informed that the Portaloo had been deposited exactly at the grid reference submitted. It seemed that the RAF and the German army use a slightly different grid system. Ever sticklers for rules, our German colleagues required that the existing Portaloo be taken directly back to their camp, another grid reference had to be submitted, then the item would be delivered to the correct position. This took all day. The NCO in charge wouldn't or couldn't simply pick it up from the wrong field and drop it off with us.

A few days later in the same site an anthro, who was also a senior Dutch reserve army officer, while walking to the area designated as a men's urinal strayed out of the cordon. As an amateur botanist he'd been distracted by some interesting foliage. As he walked closer to take a photograph, he'd ducked under some overhanging branches protruding from a high bush over a footpath leading to a nearby Muslim village, then became aware that a length of wire had become entangled around one of his legs. He shouted out so a German soldier made his way to him and saw what he believed to be a booby-trap tripwire coiled around his leg. With the aid of another soldier this was safely disentangled. It was found to have originally been attached to a Mills grenade which they found hidden in the bush directly above where our Dutch buddy had stood. The wire was still attached to the grenade, but thankfully was broken elsewhere. Once we left the site that afternoon, the soldiers blew it up. It was still active. We knew from experience that it was commonplace for the military forces who carried out these atrocities to leave booby traps in the hope of killing more of their enemy as they returned to check on their relatives or properties. The small path here was a cut-through between two Muslim villages that were quite close together, a fact probably known to those who laid the trap. This was undeniably a very lucky escape for our Dutchman and a bloody good reminder to all of us of the danger of live ordnance all around us (see photo plate section).

Chapter 40

Fatal Bombing of the UN HQ Building in Baghdad

When my mobile phone rang in August 2003 I was hoping it was an invitation to some social function. Not so. The caller was actually my good friend and former Met colleague Bill Gent with whom I had worked on many a surveillance operation while in the Flying Squad and who was my team leader on the Met's first 'Crimestoppers' project. Bill had retired from the Met and was now in charge of global security for UNICEF based in New York. He'd been summoned to the office of former Met ACC Dave Veness (now Sir David) who was Under Secretary-General for Safety and Security at the United Nations, effectively the head of security for all UN agencies worldwide. It was thought that a suicide bomber had exploded a device while driving a lorry into the UN HQ Building in Baghdad, Iraq some time earlier, causing the deaths of twenty-two UN staff including the UN Secretary-General's Special Representative, Sérgio Vieira de Mello, a vastly experienced UN diplomat. Mr Veness wanted a suitably experienced forensic examiner to conduct an investigation on behalf of UN interests separate to the enquiry to be undertaken by the military. Both knew of my past as a Met Lab Sgt which is why my name cropped up and Bill contacted me. It was an added bonus that I was also now a UN staff member with the ICTY in The Hague.

With some reservations I eventually agreed to go to Baghdad. Out of respect I spoke with the ICTY Head of Investigations who agreed to release me for this important task after asking me if I was sure what I would be going in to. Someone had to do it, so why not me? Arrangements were swiftly made and after several emails and phone calls I was on a fairly small UN jet approaching Baghdad Airport a day later. As the airport came into view, the pilot announced that due to anticipated turbulence he would have to corkscrew the plane steeply to land. At this I saw a couple of military helicopters rapidly ascending on either side of us with silver paper-like strips streaming out of their open doors. I had enough military awareness to know that this was 'chaff': small strips of aluminium foil used to deter missiles by obstructing radar detection. Was I glad to land?! Convoyed to a central Baghdad hotel which was pretty basic with little security apparent, I met other members of this UN investigation team. The team leader was a former Canadian army officer; the expo was an ex-Australian army officer; a former Met solicitor was the legal expert; a former Met sergeant who was now a security officer within the UN (with whom I would again work closely in the not-too-distant future when we both held other UN security posts in Sudan) and yours truly as the forensic investigator made up this motley crew. None of us knew one another, but it soon became obvious that each was an expert in their field so we bonded quickly.

As soon as was practicable we took a look at the bombed UN building where I made myself known to an FBI counter-terrorism team investigating the incident who were present at the scene when we arrived. The FBI team was led by a Special Agent who for reasons of security I will refer to as 'Dave' (not his real name). He and his impressive colleagues had the investigation well in hand and they very kindly agreed to share their findings with me and the rest of the UN team. This was a bonus. Having worked with the FBI before, I'd found that they were not always so liberal with their data. It was agreed that I would accompany them on their day-to-day enquiries starting the following morning. I was to make my way to their base at the Green Zone and take it from there. I took the opportunity to speak with members of Mr de Mello's protection team (PROT) who outlined their disappointment at the reduction of security brought about by their charge. They also blamed themselves for his demise, which I thought bizarre. Upon my return to The Hague I spoke with a member of my team who I knew had carried out PROT work when in the British army and he confirmed that this was not unusual. No PROT member ever accepts losing their charge.

It was established that on Tuesday, 19 August at around 1630 hours the bomber had driven an orange-coloured flatbed truck up a side road off Canal Road, central Baghdad to a point directly underneath the office of the Special Representative, which implied some insider knowledge, then the explosive devices and assorted ordnance carried in the vehicle were set off. The blast damage was enormous. The impact crater was 3.5 metres in diameter and 1.5 metres deep. The FBI team estimated that approximately 1,000kg of explosives had been involved.

Orange-painted vehicles are the property of the Baghdad local authority, so Dave's team wanted to attend the authority's office and see if one was missing. I could cause them a problem because of my UN kit, advised Dave. Wearing a UN light blue helmet and matching bulletproof vest was tantamount to giving a sniper an extremely good target. Dave was concerned that I was unarmed too. Once he realized that I'd been weapon-trained in the Met, we went to a firing range in the Green Zone where I became conversant with an automatic pistol and rifle which I carried when out with the Feds. I swapped my helmet and vest for a US camouflaged version as well. This was all comforting, believe me. Nearly everyone in Baghdad in the heat of the summer wears a form of long robe under which anything can be hidden. This makes one a trifle nervous when on foot, which sometimes was the only mode of travel for us. Our enquiries ascertained that the lorry had been stolen several days before the incident from a local authority yard.

Back at the scene we painstakingly sifted through considerable debris, eventually discovering a partial human hand, still with a couple of fingers attached, which was taped to part of a steering wheel. It appeared that our bomber may not have been entirely happy to volunteer for martyrdom:

- Had he feared his determination would leave him, therefore he secured himself to the steering wheel?
- Had the device been remotely set off by another's hand?

Two feet and partial legs (right and left), a single portion of a human spine, other parts of both right and left hands and one ear were recovered in a forensic sweep conducted over a 75m stretch from the left side of the point of impact. No body parts were found in a similar sweep to the right of the point of contact, which led us to confirm that only the driver was in the cabin when the explosion occurred, the body being blown out of the driver's door area. DNA swabs were taken from the inside of the truck's cabin for comparison with the recovered body parts.

Dave and I interviewed as many of the injured victims as we could within the hospital facility in the Green Zone and managed to locate the only eye-witness to this awful bombing. This was a young local woman who was visiting her sister (a UN employee) and heard the sound of a speeding lorry with a high-revving engine outside her sister's office window. She saw and heard small stone chippings thrown up by this vehicle rattle on the outside glass of the window. When she looked out to see what was happening, she noticed an orange flatbed lorry with a brown cabin crash into the security wall of the building further up the road and was then knocked unconscious by a blast. Another UN employee in the same office was logging off from her computer, which was recorded as being at 1624 hours.

After a couple of weeks in Baghdad, unnerving at times due to the distinct absence of sufficient security in my opinion for our team's members, we thankfully withdrew to a safer place in order to compile the report required by Mr Veness. Undeniably without the extremely valuable assistance of Dave and his team this would have been much less in detail and content. We had expected to be housed in the military stronghold and former Gaddafi palace now known as the Green Zone, but this was not to be. Instead we were booked into a rather shabby, cheap hotel with the only visible security being a not-so-young gent in robes who sat and often slept on a bench at the front of the premises armed with one of the oldest Kalashnikov semi-automatic rifles I'd ever seen. As a result, we spent as much time as possible in the Green Zone or at the crime scene. In my case I had the reassurance of carrying a firearm while I was engaged with the Feds. Unfortunately I had to leave it with them when I returned to our hotel rooms. Undeniably this was the most troubling and disconcerting period in my experience as far as personal security was concerned. It was way outside my comfort zone.

Shortly before the bombing, Mr de Mello had asked the Australian and US military to remove their roadblocks which stood just outside the UN building and because of complaints from some UN staff members also barred the military from using their canteen facilities, citing that weapons should not be carried within UN buildings and the presence of military personnel diminished the UN's impartiality. It was no coincidence that very soon after these decisions were made, the bomber struck. Furthermore, had it not been for the swift reaction of the very same Australian and US military encamped nearby who rushed to the scene, rendered first aid and called in helicopters to airlift survivors to medical facilities within the Green Zone, the loss of life would have been much greater.

Ironically, parked in the yard compound of the UN building were two South African-made 'Wolf' armoured vehicles that could have been utilized as ambulances, nicknamed 'Wolf' because of the V-shaped front aspect of the radiator, headlamps and bumpers that resemble a wolf's face. These vehicles were expressly built to withstand land mines but because of their acknowledged high fuel consumption, a decision had been made not to use them or even park them fuelled and ready for any emergency in Baghdad. I'd seen them in use clearing grave sites in Kosovo in 1999 and was impressed with their capability. The South African military used them successfully in large numbers as APCs.

I ensured that these findings were outlined in our Baghdad report and as a result was subsequently asked by UN HQ New York to contact the global Head of Security at UN WFP (World Food Programme) in Rome, Mick Lorentzen, who had a few months earlier submitted a paper highlighting the lack of ambulance facilities within UN buildings in parts of the world where there was no equivalent facility. With ICTY permission I spent a week in Rome at WFP HQ working with Mick, a former Royal Marine officer, as we put together a more detailed report for the consideration of the UN to equip and supply such vehicles as and where required. With the invaluable advice and practical assistance of Italian medical doctor Dr Sergio Arena, also a WFP staff member, we decided on several options of type and size of vehicle and the sort of basic to more advanced first-aid equipment each could carry. A few months later they both joined me in London where we booked into a hotel for a couple of days to work out the finer details of our recommendations which had received a very positive reaction from senior New York WFP staff. Dr Arena even had meticulously-detailed plans drawn up showing the interior layouts of several suitable vehicles. One was a Land Rover Defender, but of the others I'm afraid my memory is vague. More than likely they'd be European makes such as VW, Citroën or Fiat.

Back in Rome our hard-won detailed Revised Concept Paper, as the report was now named, was eventually finalized, incorporating photographs and diagrams, costings, and recommendations of senior WFP and other UN agency chiefs and submitted for due consideration to UN HQ New York. For reasons best known to a few senior New York staffers, it hasn't been implemented. Given the vast amounts of money I'm aware the UN wastes annually, the cost of purchasing, equipping and installing such emergency vehicles worldwide would be small change. Notwithstanding the cost compared to the potential for saving lives, it's a no-brainer.

Chapter 41

UNICEF in Sudan

It was a wet and miserable day in The Hague when Bill Gent phoned me for a second time in so many years, this time to sound me out and offer me a job. He told me that UNICEF were about to form their largest ever humanitarian mission in Sudan and Bill considered me more than suitable for the post of Senior Security Advisor to the UNICEF Country Director. I'd no experience in that field but he was of the opinion that I could with training turn my hand to it; after all, I'd taken on the role of office manager in the then brand-new to the UK 'Crimestoppers' project which was a step into the dark for the both of us. I did fancy a bit of sun, I must admit. I liked what UNICEF was about and what they did, so once I'd read through the blurb that Bill forwarded me I was even more convinced about getting involved.

After some soul-searching I thought I'd give it a go. I flew to New York at UNICEF's expense to discuss matters further. Some days later I committed myself to UNICEF, so upon my return to The Hague I submitted my resignation to the ICTY. I knew the Evidence Unit would be in great hands as I took steps to ensure that my deputy, former Royal Military Police sergeant Geraldine 'Gerry' Thatcher would take over. Gerry organized the most remarkable leaving party I've ever attended, never mind been the recipient of. It was a truly amazing evening attended by the many friends and colleagues I'd worked with over the past five years. One of the highlights was a trial attorney from Botswana, where he claimed to be minor royalty, singing Frank Sinatra's ballad *My Way* to me. He had a good voice. It was quite moving, actually.

I spent a week on a UN security officer's basic training course in Cairo, then flew to Khartoum where I'd be based. The UNICEF compound there is a large converted villa with a couple of outhouses, one of which contained a staff café and the other I selected as my office because it was slightly apart from the main building and positioned near the main entrance. I was issued with my own UN radio-equipped vehicle. The Country Director was an experienced diplomat and we got on well from the start. My main task was to liaise with all other UN security chiefs in Sudan and security personnel in the embassies to keep up to date with the banditry, proxy fighting and general turmoil throughout this troubled country. I had responsibility for more than 100 international staff and another 400 natively-recruited personnel stationed at several UNICEF compounds throughout Sudan and South Sudan.

I rented a small and thankfully fully air-conditioned first-storey apartment not far from the international airport. Power cuts were a regular nuisance and it took me a while to get used to the call to prayer initiated by a muezzin from a nearby minaret five times a day, the earliest being at sunrise. My landlord originally came from Nubia in the north of Sudan near the border with Egypt, famous for its pyramids and male wrestling. He was a pharmaceutical salesman (no, that's not posh for drug dealer) who imported medical products for hospitals and pharmacies. He and his family occupied the ground floor. His young son would often pop in to practise his English on me and a neighbour Glenn Gilbertson, a retired Met Det Supt who was commissioner of the UN Police Unit in Sudan.

I engaged a young Eritrean refugee as a maid who often brought her sister with her. Everyone has a maid in Khartoum. They were obliged to wear full Arabic robes when moving around the city, but once inside they'd discard these and go about their work in jeans, flip-flops and modern tops, listening to pop music. Despite having experienced a great deal of unpleasantness and victimization in their young lives, they always had a smile on their faces and strived to make the best of what they had. Their father had been imprisoned in Eritrea and they had no idea if he was alive or dead. Their brother was conscripted into the army and they didn't know where he was either. Happily, soon afterwards they were granted citizen entry to Canada where they've completed university degrees and started new lives.

In the summer Sudan is prone to haboobs. These are extremely strong winds that pick up desert sand and advance at speed, raining the sand over everything in their path. One afternoon I was completing some paperwork in my flat after the maids had cleaned it and left when the landlord's son rushed in crying out 'Haboob coming.' He checked the windows and veranda doors were closed, then pointed towards the airport where I saw the amazing sight of the entire sky embroiled in a dark red sandstorm heading our way. As it drew nearer it became darker and darker and the noise level louder and louder. When it struck the house I thought the windows would smash. Luckily they didn't; however, sand was blowing in through every nook and cranny and believe me, in a Sudanese-built house there are lots of nooks and crannies. It took several minutes to pass while we stood in pitch darkness in the middle of the day. You'll not be surprised to learn that these storms are often the cause of loss of life, especially if one's caught out in the open. When light returned, my entire apartment was coated in a layer of fine red sand. So much for the maid's good efforts.

No staff member could travel anywhere without security clearance and in order for them to obtain that I needed to be assured that the journey was necessary and that the mode and route proposed were safe. Thankfully the UK, German, Dutch, American, Japanese and Italian embassy security staff were willing to share their Intel with me. They also shared their bar facilities, which was even better given that Sudan is a Sharia country where alcohol is banned. Obviously there's always a way to get behind this ban, but it was easier for all to attend a legally permitted bar than get involved in the black market. In fairness, the Sudanese authorities were quite lax with internationals obtaining the odd bottle of spirits or whatever. Security officers from all the other agencies soon became buddies; after all, we were all in this together, so at least twice a week we would congregate to exchange Intel and the odd tipple.

I'd accompany one or two of them on visits in-country to check various UN compounds and speak with local staff to check the safety of routes to these compounds from Khartoum. When I toured UNICEF compounds in both Sudan and South Sudan I'd often be accompanied by a WFP, UNHCR or other UN agency security officer. My deputy Sidahmed Akood was a former Sudan army intelligence officer who was well-connected. His father had been an army general and an uncle a DCS in the Sudan police when Sudan was under colonial rule. I met this uncle during a visit to a nearby UN compound with Sid (my nickname for him, which he liked as it sounded like CID). He was proud to show me a photograph of him in police uniform attending a colonial officers' course at Bramshill Police College in the UK. Bramshill was a staff training establishment for senior police officers in England and Wales until 2015.

Sid was very much my right-hand man, guide and trusted advisor for the two years I was with UNICEF in his country. He was also most helpful when we selected newly-trained locals as security guards to protect the compounds, warehouses and other UNICEF properties. He and I carried out quite a few sorties to Darfur refugee camps in which UNICEF had a major stake. To do this we drove two or three Jeep convoys of several days' duration during which we'd overnight in a UNICEF compound en route. To my inexperienced eye we just drove through miles and miles of sand, but the local drivers were actually following hard-to-see (for me anyway) ancient camel routes that they knew by heart. We often came across broken-down, heavily overladen and aged trucks, many of British manufacture like Bedford, for example, when we'd stop to check if the drivers needed any help. They seldom did. Overburdened donkeys and camels were commonplace. Such journeys can be a bit soporific but Sid and the local drivers lessened the tedium of these long journeys with tales of what Sudan had been like under British rule. The sight of thousands of wild camels roaming in the middle of these desert routes was awesome. Similarly, occasionally crossing paths with nomadic herdsmen was a fascinating sight. Where relevant, and due to Sid's many travels in certain regions during his army career, he'd cause us to deviate course slightly so that he could show me an old water pump or similar example of Victorian engineering which he was proud to point out had been installed by the British army or British civil engineers and still worked, not like the Chinese-built equivalents now installed, he'd say.

I was in Scotland, Aberdeen in fact, on R&R aware that Sid was about to become a father when my wife and I passed a statue of Gordon of Khartoum, or Chinese Gordon as he's also famously known, so given the historic link with this heroic Victorian soldier who was murdered by the Mahdi's dervishes in Khartoum in 1885 we popped into Marks & Spencer and bought a few items for the baby which went down a treat, especially when I mentioned the link with Gordon. On other occasions we flew by UN helicopter which was also interesting and of course effective in time-saving but not so educational. The other downside to these flights was that the machines were not exactly state of the art, so the journey was less than comfortable and very noisy even when wearing ear defenders. Other trips in small fixed-wing aircraft were far safer and allowed one to get on with some of the extensive paperwork on which the UN thrives.

UNICEF is dedicated to providing clean drinking water as well as the education of females who in turn will educate their children. UNICEF engineers sunk deep bores to obtain water sources and schools were built and staffed to educate children in some of the remotest parts of the country. A nomadic school was set up which followed herdsmen, breaking camp and setting up as they did. Goodwill ambassadors would be brought in at times to promote UNICEF's work worldwide and help generate the necessary and considerable funds needed to pay for these vitally important and life-saving tasks.

The most notable of the latter was American actress Mia Farrow who, on several occasions, I accompanied on visits to Darfur camps. She impressed me with her breadth of knowledge concerning women's rights and keenness to promote the particular plight of these poor women and children evidenced by the empathy and humanity she displayed when talking with them. I was also present once when she confronted and challenged the relevant wali (government representative responsible for a given landward area) and senior military and police officers who were responsible for the protection of these vulnerable women who were being raped and abused inside the camps or while gathering firewood nearby by the so-called guards under their command. Ms Farrow still carries out this sterling work and must have generated hundreds of thousands of dollars for UNICEF coffers over the years.

As tensions grew and armed insurgency was a possibility by those opposing the president, the security of all UN compounds needed firming up. President Omar al-Bashir had wrested power from the civil government in 1989 when as a brigadier in the Sudan army he led a military coup d'état. The old villa UNICEF called HQ was three storeys high and the material used in its original construction and later extensions made it highly flammable. The Khartoum fire brigade I'm sorry to say was shambolic, so reliance upon them in the case of a fire was low to non-existent. One UNICEF team leader had worked for an architect and drew up first-class plans for a metal fire escape. A local private fire and security firm cast an eye over these plans and gave them the thumbs-up, then after much wrangling I obtained funding to have it built. Several meetings with representatives of all staff members finalized its construction when at the same time fire-proof safes, exit doors, emergency lighting and an alarm system were installed.

Shortly after completion, and with the permission of the Country Director, I tested the system with a fire drill which every staff member had been taught during the construction period. I stood, stopwatch in hand, with a clipboard containing the names of all staff in the building, checking them off as they arrived at the RVP. Quite a few were missing so I sent a couple of security guards in to check. The result of their walk-through was that all staff on the ground floor and nearly all on the second floor had left. The ones that remained inside were Sudanese female staff. On the top floor none of the Sudanese female staff had left the building. I immediately chaired a debriefing with all staff where I learned that no Sudanese female would descend a stepladder while men stood below. Of the numerous local female staff members who'd attended the preparatory meetings and fire escape drills, none had mentioned this before. It was a combination of modesty and culture. By way of compromise, an extension to the fire escape was constructed for the use of females only which led to a separate RVP. A fire drill carried out once this was in situ was still not 100 per cent but a great deal better. Fortunately during my two-year tenure we didn't have a fire. Sudan tested my patience a lot at times but this was paid back with dividends at other times.

I also had responsibility for our staff in Juba, the capital of South Sudan, although we had an excellent security team there consisting of former New Zealand and Brazilian army officers. The latter replaced me when I left Khartoum. Juba was totally different to Khartoum. In Sudan nearly all locals wear robes, the men in white, and the ladies a bit more colourful with their heads covered. South Sudan is a Christian country so the women are not required to dress as in the Arabic north. On Sundays the kids wore their Sunday best on their way to church, the little girls charming in their pleated hair tied up with bright ribbons and even more colourful frocks. It felt almost like R&R when I was there on UNICEF business.

There was another amazing American lady with whom I had the pleasure of spending some time in Wau (pronounced 'Wow'), a small town on the western bank of the River Jur some 400 miles north of Juba, the capital of South Sudan. In my opinion, certainly in the early 2000s, Wau was the absolute pits of this new but extremely impoverished country. The lady in question was a self-styled millionaire, as was her husband, who resided with their sons in the borough of Manhattan in New York City, USA where she was an entrepreneur and philanthropist.

Over the years she'd donated tens of thousands of dollars to UNICEF and it was an honour to escort her to this awful place in order for her to see a school and fresh water facility that had been set up using some of her funding. The UNICEF Special Representative was called away at short notice so couldn't accompany us. We flew there in a not-too-comfortable UN plane to the nearest airstrip, then via an even less comfortable UN helicopter to the UNICEF compound in which we would spend the evening before visiting the school the following day.

The local UNICEF team leader turned up with some light refreshments and an apology for the lack of amenities in the compound which consisted of two linked Portakabins, only one of which was fitted with air conditioning. The toilet was a hole in the ground (typical in Sudan), with a grid atop surrounded by hessian screening, situated about 100 metres away. Nearby at a large bivouac attached to a Mercedes Jeep we were introduced to two German pilots who used the compound when in the area. They were watching a football match featuring Germany v Italy on a portable TV being run from the Jeep's battery and invited us to join them with a few cold beers. Luxury. We accepted and I spent the next half an hour or so trying to explain the rules of soccer to this lovely American lady. Not easy. At the same time she was learning German expletives every time a foul was committed on a German player or when they missed scoring a goal.

At the end of the game we thanked the pilots for their hospitality and, after making sure the lady's air-con was operating, I went to my own room which was broiling and, most annoyingly, although equipped with air-con it had not been linked up to the power supply yet, to try to get some much-needed sleep. Due to the ever-present threat of malaria-bearing mosquitoes I couldn't open any windows either. I soon heard a knock on my door. It was my American charge who was a bit wary of the terrain and the dark and wished me to accompany her to the toilet area. Adopting my Sir Galahad pose I did so, then with eyes averted and whistling to let her know I wouldn't be listening, stood guard a short way off. We laughed about this when local staff collected us the following morning. She was very much impressed with the school and water facility and easily engaged with the young female students, some of whom were from the nomadic community, asking them what they wanted to achieve in their future lives and discussing with their teachers what their needs were, all the while distributing pencils, jotters and other stationery goods she'd brought with her as gifts.

222

Bidding goodbye to my UNICEF colleagues, we caught the helicopter to the nearest reasonably-sized airport where my companion had arranged for her private jet to collect us for the flight to Khartoum. I'd never flown in a Lear jet before, so it was a bit of a treat to say the least. Absolute comfort. (I want one!) During this extremely pleasant flight she confided in me that occasionally when traffic was gridlocked in Manhattan she couldn't rely on their private chauffeur but rather used their private helicopter to take their sons to school. I was impressed and more than a little amazed that a lady with such a lifestyle had put up with such an unpleasantly smelly drop toilet in the open and a very basic Portakabin bedroom without complaint, notwithstanding the creditable work her regular and handsome donations had allowed UNICEF to carry out. It was truly an honour meeting her.

My sister contacted me at around this time with the sad news that my mother had been rushed to hospital and was unlikely to live much longer. Pancreatic cancer had been diagnosed. She was 84 years young. After taking a couple of very frustrating days getting home from the Sudan, I drove up to St Margaret's Hospital in Dunfermline, Fife and was lucky to have a day with her and my sister as Mum came in and out of a morphine-induced coma. She was in a side room on her own and was attended by a wonderful NHS team. The young female doctor explained Mum's situation to us and waived visiting times so that we could remain with her at our pleasure.

I remember asking mum if there was anything that she wanted, to which she replied that she'd like a tub of vanilla ice cream. I popped out and bought a carton in the hospital shop and when I was spooning it to her she asked me if I remembered her doing this for me when I was a bairn (Scots for child). I found that very touching. She went on to enjoy three further cartons that day. Gradually her periods of lucidity shortened and her heartbeat and breathing altered. I recall holding her hand, my sister held the other, and with a tear in my eye told her it was ok if she wanted to leave us now. All would be fine. She'd brought us both up well. Shortly after that her life spark went out and I knew I was holding the hand of a deceased person. Her soul had gone and her whole body seemed to relax and be at peace. I shall be forever grateful to these fine nurses, doctors and other NHS staff who cared so very well for my mum in her last days. It was also cathartic for me to be there with her when she died. I knew then what I'd missed by not having this opportunity with my beloved grandfather.

When I returned to Khartoum after a short break I learned that two of our international female staff members were on a mission to a UNICEF compound when it was raided by the Sudan Religious Police. These units, as their name implies, ensure that Muslims do not transgress Sharia law. In this instance they claimed that alcohol was kept on the premises and that it was being offered to and drunk by national Muslim staff, a big no-no in UNICEF. A number of individuals were taken into custody including our two ladies, during which time one of them was allegedly sexually assaulted by a police officer in a police detention room. After release without charge, she complained to her UNICEF chain of management. When they returned to Khartoum I spoke with them both and established what had happened. The director then decided, with other UN agency leaders, to send a selected team to that compound to investigate the allegation. I volunteered to lend my expertise. This was politely refused on the basis that I may be seen as too confrontational because of my Scotland Yard background. I argued that as the Sudan police had been trained in British police methods, with my knowledge of what records they were obliged to maintain, for example staff allocation in the detention room on the day in question, I should be able to pinpoint if not the actual officer but the few who were assigned to the task at the time, thus minimizing the team's time and efforts. It was not to be.

No staff member with a law enforcement background was chosen. I surreptitiously briefed a member of this team as to what to ask the O/I/C of the Sudan police station in question and gave a few pointers as to how to direct the enquiry where possible. Suffice to say no-one was identified as being responsible for this insidious assault. In fairness UNICEF did supply support and assistance to the unfortunate staff member, but I feel that a more robust attitude should have been adopted from the start. In agreement with me was my colleague Sid who suggested he and I go it alone on a follow-up visit. Good idea though it was, I knew it would not be acceptable to the director. Diplomacy was never my forte.

My long-suffering partner, best friend, confidante and wife Sheila, herself a former Met DS with Anti-Terrorist Branch experience, joined me in my second year in the Sudan after she retired from the police. Sheila had looked forward to joining me in The Hague where we had many friends, and she envisaged 'doing lunch' and maybe partaking of the odd game of tennis with the ladies there. All that went out the window when I accepted the UNICEF post. At a team leaders' meeting one day I was asked by a child protection unit leader who'd met Sheila and knew she'd been a police officer if she had any experience in their particular line of work. Suffice to say she had and was soon interviewed and offered a six-month contract. She became involved with a Family and Child Protection Unit set up within the Sudan police. This ground-breaking unit was made up of police investigators, social workers and child psychologists with the express intention of investigating crimes and abuse of women and children utilizing the principles of the Scandinavian Barnahus system. This is where victims are interviewed outside of police stations in a safe house with soft furnishings, where interviews are videoed and support is offered to the victim. The aim was to train local personnel to conduct these investigations and remove the burden from UNICEF and other UN agencies. A necessary and most worthy task which resulted in her being granted a further contract of seven months' duration.

While I was involved in the Baghdad bombing investigation my good lady had been attached to the British Embassy in Kabul, Afghanistan, assisting with the investigation of two former war lords who'd been arrested working in a London restaurant by Anti-Terrorist Branch officers and charged with war crimes in Afghanistan. Sheila's task was to interview the female victims who'd been kidnapped, raped and held as sex slaves, then passed on to other war lords when replaced by younger girls who were similarly kidnapped and held by these vile criminals. The women gave video evidence which was transmitted in real time to the trial court at the Old Bailey in the City of London from the embassy. Sheila and I met up for a bit of joint R&R in Dubai at this time. We've often wondered if anyone there overheard our conversations during several restaurant meals when we discussed my working in Iraq and Sheila elaborating on her Afghanistan experiences; how weird we must have sounded to them.

Chapter 42

Historical Enquiries Team (HET), part of the Police Service Northern Ireland (PSNI)

After several months of retirement, catching up with some long overdue DIY tasks, a spot of gardening and regular walks with our two spaniels Dylan & Max, I was getting a little bored so I updated my CV and chucked it into the ether to see if there were any part-time posts I could pick up. Quite soon thereafter I received a telephone call from a group that sought employment for retired police officers asking me if I knew anything about the Historical Enquiries Team (HET) within the Police Service of Northern Ireland (PSNI) which was currently recruiting retired police detectives, particularly those with specialist skills. I didn't, so they sent me an email with details of this organization. In 2005 Sir Hugh Orde, OBE, QPM as the then Commissioner of the PSNI, a widely-respected and experienced senior high flyer, convinced the Northern Ireland house of government at Stormont that an independent body should be set up to investigate the numerous murders that had been committed during the Troubles which, for a variety of reasons, had not been properly investigated at the time. HET was the result.

The substantial brief that HET was given was to conduct cold-case reviews on 3,268 deaths from 2,516 incidents that occurred in Northern Ireland during the Troubles from January 1969 until the Good Friday Agreement in 1998. At its height 175 staff were engaged, the majority being seasoned murder investigators from all over the UK, selected military experts and civilian specialists plus an invaluable team of ex-RUC detectives, most of whom had personal knowledge of many of the incidents under review. The RUC preceded the PSNI as the civilian police authority in Northern Ireland.

A couple of days later I attended a brief Monday morning interview at Stansted Airport with two former Met senior detectives – one had been

226

a DCS and the other a Det Supt – neither of whom I had met before, as they awaited their weekly flight to Belfast. They didn't know me either but were aware of the role of the Met LLO which was a post they wanted at HET where both had been engaged for some time. I felt this was an extremely worthwhile opportunity to help bring some closure to the grief of the relatives of the many victims of gunmen from both sides of the conflict so I signed up to HET. I'd already discussed the possibility with my wife, who agreed it was a job to which I could lend my expertise. For the next five years I'd fly back and forth from Gatwick to Belfast on Mondays and Fridays, as did most of my colleagues, to carry out this important work. I set up a Forensic Desk for HET and with almost daily contact with Dr Ruth Griffin, OBE, a leading biologist at the Forensic Service Northern Ireland (FSNI) laboratory and her dedicated team of another female biologist and a civil servant we searched the records of each of the 3,268 deaths HET re-investigated and reviewed any forensic evidence still in existence to see if it could be re-examined, given the advances of forensic science since 1968. No mean feat, I can tell you.

One of the almost daily routines I had to get used to was running a mirror underneath my private car to ensure that nothing untoward had been suspended there overnight. Given that I'd worked in a number of war zones, it felt incongruous carrying out this function in a part of the UK. Frequently changing routes from my rented accommodation to the HET offices also reminded me of the hazards of working in this capacity in Northern Ireland. Watching your Ps and Qs while socializing was another constant. All of this apart, it was a great place to be and I found a good many cultural locations as well as restaurants and pubs where I enjoyed the fare and the company. Belfast especially offers a very interesting and pleasant range of social events.

With a former RUC colleague or two every PSNI station was contacted requesting that they search their property and evidence stores and let us know if they held any items or evidence pertinent to these cases. When we received a positive response we'd collect same and bring it back to the HET office just outside Lisburn where we'd discuss with the relevant enquiry team leader and Dr Griffin what, if anything, could be done forensically. This brought about the recovery of firearms, ballistic items, bullets, clothing, blood swabs and a hoard of other items, most of which had previously been through the FSNI Lab process but some of which had not. During the Troubles the RUC were not able to carry out detailed forensic crime scene examinations that police in other parts of the UK could. Furthermore, items were lost in police stations that were subject to explosive or mortar attack. Reading through the many detailed dossiers and witness statements produced as a result of the 2,516 incidents, my respect for the way in which the RUC carried out their duties under fire increased incrementally.

For reasons of sub judice (being under judgement), coupled with the fact that PSNI and other law enforcement agencies are still continuing enquiries into many perpetrators of these crimes, I'm not able to describe the nature of many of the incidents looked into by the HET. One case I can mention is where a gunman was brought to justice after the FSNI detected DNA in cigarette stubs and spent bullet cartridges recovered from the murder of a young off-duty RUC constable. The officer had returned to his private car in the car park of Victoria Hospital, Belfast having visited his wife who'd just given birth to their first child. The gunman shot him at close range in the back of his head. The gunman was arrested by PSNI officers and convicted at trial for murder. Frustratingly, because of the Good Friday Agreement he could only receive a two-year prison sentence. This conviction was only possible because of the advances of forensic science.

The only other case I shall highlight was where colleagues were able to inform a former member of the British army who served in Belfast during the Troubles that an FSNI ballistic re-examination of bullets fired from his issued rifle compared with one removed from the body of a 7-year-old girl at post mortem proved that his weapon had not fired the fatal shot. The unfortunate little girl had been playing with friends in the street when IRA gunmen hiding nearby opened fire on an army foot patrol. The soldiers returned fire and she was tragically caught in the crossfire. A flawed RMP investigation at the time found, incorrectly, that this squaddie, then a mere 19 years of age, had fired the shot. The ex-soldier, now in his mid 60s, broke down in tears when told. He had carried the grief and blame for this wee girl's death for his entire adult life.

During the five years that I was a part of the HET team I met and worked with many remarkable investigators and forensic scientists as well as enjoying the friendliness of the people in 'Norern Iron'. Over that period the HET carried out cold-case reviews on each and every case twice to ensure no stone was left unturned, but continually suffered criticism from various sections of the community who were dissatisfied with the return, some because of their political bias. Allegations that HET investigators adopted a 'softly, softly' approach when interviewing former police or army personnel abounded, which were completely untrue and without reason. All interviewees were treated in exactly the same manner. At the end of 2013 cutbacks reduced capability somewhat and the director, a former Met Commander, resigned, as did his deputy, the former head of CID in Greater Manchester Police. Both were well-respected, prominent and very experienced detectives.

The new PSNI Commissioner decided that two former UK police officers now serving in the PSNI should replace them. With the best of intentions and no doubt the professionalism and determination these officers would bring to the post, they were not career detectives and did not have the depth of experience in dealing with the nature and number of murders being dealt with by the HET. One of the initial major policy decisions made by them was to review all cases once more. This would mean a third time for me.

Letters were sent out to all relatives of the many victims who had engaged with the HET informing them of this decision and the fact that as a direct result the process they were now part of would be reviewed and this would cause substantial delay. After a great deal of soul-searching I decided this was no longer for me. If the cases were to be reviewed yet again, then fresh eyes and minds should do so. With regret I resigned and with a heavy heart a few weeks later drove my car onto the Stena Line ferry to Scotland. Within nine months the PSNI, as a result of pressure and the withdrawal of funding from Stormont, pulled the plug on the HET which left hundreds of families of the many victims of these crimes with no closure; a diabolical state of affairs.

Chapter 43

Remembering Srebrenica

In September 2016 I was immensely proud and privileged to be a member of a delegation of former PHR and UN forensic experts invited back to Sarajevo on behalf of the charity 'Remembering Srebrenica'. I was truly amazed and pleased at the advances of scientific DNA identification spearheaded by the International Commission on Missing Persons (ICMP) which carries on this vital identification work, which was started by us in 1996, to this day. The rejuvenation of the region, plus the hopes and aspirations of many Bosniaks we spoke with, was reassuring too. Obviously a lot has still to be accomplished and the recent past will never be forgotten, but with hard work, patience and goodwill a great deal could and should be achieved.

This trip was brought about because of the organizational efforts of former mortuary technician and fellow Scot Robert McNeil, MBE, who is also a very accomplished artist, his specialized art subject being portrayals of the work he voluntarily undertook in temporary PHR and ICTY morgues as a result of the atrocities in the former Yugoslavia. His paintings have been displayed in a number of eminent artistic venues in the UK. I worked with Robert in Bosnia in 1996 and am proud also to count him as a friend.

Especially memorable was a courageous address by one of the mothers of Srebrenica who spoke of the loss of her husband and son and how it had affected her and her daughter's lives. The determination she displayed to keep living for her grandchildren, setting up a small business selling books, flowers and mementos outside the UN Dutch Battalion military base where this all began, was as humbling as her resilience and fortitude were impressive.

Visits to the Dutch Bat base, the rather eerie Tunnel of Hope and an art gallery depicting scenes from the war in Yugoslavia known as Galerija 11/07/95 were outstanding. I noted the serenity and silence of my colleagues as we spent time in these venues, no doubt reminiscing about our presence and work there in 1996. I really do think that we did in fact make a difference (see photo plate section).

I would like for the record to praise Resad Trobonja who was not only a superb guide but a knowledgeable patriot who answered the many questions we put to him, as he vividly described his experiences and 'told it like it was' during the siege of Sarajevo when he was a teenage soldier there. It was a privilege and a pleasure meeting and talking with him.

Since that trip I've passed on details of the work of this fine charity Remembering Srebrenica via Facebook and informed the Association of ex-Scotland Yard Detectives (Ex-Tecs) about it in the hope of interesting others in the admirable work the charity carries out for the benefit of and with large numbers of relatives of the many victims of these atrocities. It is my intention to make a donation to this charity from the eventual sales of this book.

It has been extremely gratifying and a great privilege to have been involved in such important work over the years and I feel especially proud as well as fortunate to have met with and worked alongside so many competent and internationally well-respected individuals, some of whom I now count among my friends. I'm also truly pleased that some of them received appropriate recognition for their good work. For my own efforts over the years I accrued two police medals, a UN Kosovo campaign medal, a UN Kosovo medal for Services to Peacekeeping, four Commissioner's Commendations granted for various purposes including courage, detective ability, professionalism and determination for a number of murder investigations, plus two Commissioner's Commendations for my work as the BFT co-ordinator in Kosovo, as well as letters of appreciation and gratitude from the FCO, former ICTY Lead Prosecutor Judge Mrs Carla Del Ponte and her deputy Graham Blewitt, and one on behalf of the late former UN Secretary-General Kofi Annan for my participation in the investigation into the fatal bombing of the UN building in Baghdad.

Not bad for the illegitimate son of a dockyard worker who'd grown up in poky wee council accommodation throughout the less attractive of Fife villages created in the 1950s to house workers whose only opportunity of employment was the expanding coal business. Ironically, within twenty-five years the industry had shrunk beyond recognition causing redundancy after redundancy, and in many cases families had to move away to find alternative work and homes.

Tantamount in my thoughts throughout this extremely important, albeit arduous, harrowing and oft times gruesome work was a quote I'd made to a reporter or journalist very early on in my career to the effect that 'The people in these graves were not allowed a voice. It's our task to give them back that voice.' In my humble opinion we did just that.

Maybe now if my old Fife Constabulary ACC was still alive he would acknowledge, and hopefully accept, when considering all the varied and in more than a few cases rather important investigations in which I've been involved in both my police and other careers that, after all is said and done, my transfer south to the Met was indeed a good move; in fact, a very good move. Likewise my old headmaster, the formidable Mr Eadie.

In my endeavours to transmit my thoughts and feelings into this missive I sincerely hope that readers will understand what drove me throughout my professional life, and many deaths, and consider this literary work as a well-intentioned example of social history as well as a record of true crime and not simply a collection of egotistical scribblings.

Would I do it all over again? You better believe it!

Index

Annan, Kofi (former UN Secretary General), 231
Athulathmudali, Lalith (late Sri Lanka politician), 142, 146
Atkinson, Kate, 5

Baghdad, Iraq, 211–15, 225, 231
Bashir, al Omar (former President of Sudan), 220
Beath High School, Cowdenbeath, 4, 9, 32
Bevan, Aneurin 'Nye', 7
Black, Sue (Dame Professor of Anthropology), 115, 133
Blewitt, Graham, 231
Bourke, Billy (former T/DC MPS), 57
Bratunac, Kosovo, 172
Britton, Paul, 135–7
Brown, Bernie (former PC MPS), 55
Buckell, Chris, (former DS Flying Squad), 111
Bunn, John (former Commander NSY), 170, 177

Campbell, Ian, 10, 13, 42
Campbell, Irene, 10
Celina, Kosovo, 176–7

Cerska, Bosnia & Herzegovina, 158–64
Chesshyre, Robert, x, 198
Clarke, Michael (former PC West Yorkshire Police), 194, 198
Connolly, Billy, 22, 79
Cook, Robin (late UK Foreign Secretary) , 179–80
Crosby, Bing, 76–7
Crosby, Kathy, 76–7

De Mello, Sergio (late UN Special Representative for Baghdad), 211–12, 214
Dicks, GW & Sons, 3
Dragonara Cemetery, Pristina, 195
Dunbar, Adrian, 184
Dunfermline, Fife, 1, 4, 6, 8, 13–17, 34, 51, 223
Dunfermline Silk Mills, 11

Eadie, Mr (late Headmaster of Beath High School), 9, 232
Edwards, Alec (former Detective Chief Superintendent NSY), 71, 141

Farrow, Mia, 220
Fellows,Turnbull, Sheila, 224–5

Ferguson, Sir Alex, 34
Ferrira, Anthony, 128
Fischer, Herr Joschka (German
  Foreign Minister), 179
Foran, Martin, 93–4
Frik, PS Frank (Politie
  Nederlands), 154
Fulton, Billy (former RUC DS),
  192–3, 198, 201, 205

Gent, Bill (former Detective
  Superintendent NSY), 114,
  211, 216
Gilbertson, Glenn (former UN
  Police Commissioner in
  Sudan), 217
Grech, George (former
  Commissioner Malta Police),
  82–4
Green River Killer, 208
  see also Ridgway
Grieve, John (former Deputy
  Assistant Commissioner NSY),
  x, 104, 149
Griffin, Dr Ruth (former Biologist
  at Forensic Science Northern
  Ireland), 227
Gwilliam, Steve (former
  Detective Superintendent
  NSY), 188

Haglund, Bill, 152
Harris, Richard, 78
Hendon Police College,
  15, 53–4
Hogg, Quntin QC (late Lord
  Chancellor), 63
Holy Joe, 3

Imbert, Sir Peter (late
  Commissioner NSY), 78, 113

Kalesija, Bosnia & Herzegovina,
  153, 163, 168
Karadzic, Radovan, 200
Karakaj, Kosovo (see also Red
  Dam), 172
Kaunda, Didri, 188, 191
Kaunda, Kenneth (former
  President of Zambia), 188
Kaunda, Major Wezi, 188, 191
Kelly, Jack, (late DC Flying
  Squad), 106
Kerr, Bill, 61–2
Khartoum, Sudan, 216–21, 223–4
Kinnear, Mrs, 30–1, 40
Kirkcaldy, Fife, 4, 13, 17, 22, 28, 37

Locard, Dr Edmund (Locard's
  Exchange Principle), 127, 138
Lochgelly, Fife, 2–5, 20, 56
Lorentzen, Mick (World Food
  Programme [WFP]), 215
Lumley, Joanna, 184

Malta GC, 81–5
Mark, Sir Robert (late
  Commissioner NSY), 74
Mayne, Sir Richard (late
  Commissioner Scotland Yard), 78
McNeil, Robert, 230
McNeill, Jim (late PS Fife
  Constabulary), 39–40
McNeill, Jim Jnr, 40
Methil, Fife, 28–9, 30, 39, 47,
  50, 80
Milan, Italy, 81, 85

Milosevic, Slobodan, 200
Mintoff, Dom (former Prime
    Minister of Malta), 84
Mladic, General Radko, 200
Moon, Jim, (late PC Flying
    Squad), 71
Moon, Keith, 79
Muir, John (former PC Fife
    Constabulary), 51–2

Napper, Robert, 137–8
Neave, Airey, 92
Nettleton, Catherine, 192–3
Nickell, Alex, 137
Nickell, Rachel, 130–8, 141
Nowicki, Roy, 178
Nuttall, Merlyn, 125–8

O'Brien, Edward, 149–50
Ognall, His Lordship
    Mr Justice, 136
O'Mahoney, Maurice, 'Mo the
    Grass', 71
Orde, Sir Hugh (former Chief
    Constable PSNI), 226
O'Toole, Peter, 78
Outward Bound School,
    Burghead, 22–6

Pearse, John, (former DS Flying
    Squad) 'JP', 96–8, 100,
    103–104
Pedder, Keith (former DI
    MPS), 137
Peel, Sir Robert (former
    Commissioner Scotland Yard), 78
Physicians for Human Resources
    (PHR), 151–2, 158, 163, 165, 230

Pike, Lyn, 93–4
Pike, Richard, 93–4
Police Mobile Column (PMC),
    19–20
Ponte, Her Honour Judge Mrs
    Carla del (former ICTY Lead
    Prosecutor), 231
PP (former DS MPS), 130
Premadasa, Ranasinghe (late
    President of Sri Lanka),
    144–6
Pristina, Kosovo, 170, 193–5,
    204, 206
Prizren, Kosovo 170, 176

Rankin, Ian, 4
Red Dam (see also Karakaj), 172
Reed, Oliver, 78
Ressler, Robert (former Special
    Agent FBI), 115
Ridgway, Gary Leon (see also
    Green River Killer), 208
Roberts, Julie, 185
Rome, Italy, 85–6, 215

Sarajevo, Bosnia & Herzegovina,
    155, 166–8, 230–1
Scott, Andrew S (late PS Fife
    Constabulary), 14–17
Shepherd, Dr Richard, Home
    Office pathologist, 133, 141–3
Shirreff, Brigadier Richard, 204
Slinn, David (former Head of
    British Office, Pristina), 204
Smith, Angela, 202
Smith, Cliff (late DS MPS),
    117–18, 201–202
Sri Lanka, 141–6

Stagg, Colin, 135–7
Stein, Jock, 34
Stevens, Sir John (former Commissioner NSY), 192

Thatcher, Geraldine, 216
Thatcher, Margaret (late Prime Minister), 93
Thaw, John, 67, 74
Tito, Josip Broz (late President of Yugoslavia), 156
Trobonja, Resad, 231
Tulliallan Castle, 27, 46, 53
Turnbull, Ceri, 95, 196–7
Turnbull, Lorna, 76, 80
Tuzla, Bosnia & Herzegovina, 152, 154, 163

Vagrancy Act of 1824, 61
Veerakumar, Kulaveerasingam, 146

Velika Krusa, Kosovo, 176, 179
Veness, Sir David (former Assistant Commissioner Crime NSY), 192, 211, 214
Vukovar, Croatia, 165–9

Waterman, Dennis, 67, 74
Watts, Steve (former Detective Chief Superintendent Hants Police), 192, 198
Waldron, Sir John (late Commissioner NSY), 63
Waxwing, HMS, 8
West, Dr Iain, (late Home Office pathologist), 149
White, Chalky, (former PC Flying Squad), 96–8
Worsley, Michael QC, 72

Zambia, 188–91